W0050589

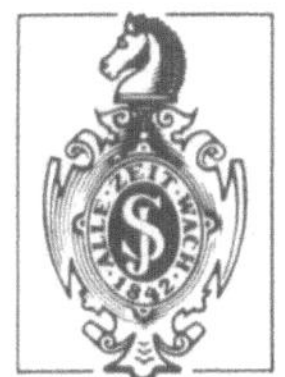

Sensory Disorders of the Bladder and Urethra

Edited by
N. J. R. George and J. A. Gosling

Foreword by Professor N. J. Blacklock

With 64 Figures

Springer-Verlag
Berlin Heidelberg New York Toyko

N. J. R. George, FRCS
Lecturer and Senior Registrar in Urology,
University Hospital of South Manchester,
Manchester M20 8LR, England

J. A. Gosling, MB, ChB, MD
Professor of Anatomy, Medical School,
University of Manchester, Oxford Road,
Manchester M13 9PT, England

ISBN-13: 978-1-4471-1394-2 e-ISBN-13: 978-1-4471-1392-8
DOI: 10.1007/978-1-4471-1392-8

Library of Congress Cataloging-in-Publication Data
Main entry under title:
Sensory disorders of the bladder and urethra.
Includes bibliographies and index. 1. Bladder – Diseases. 2. Urethra – Diseases. 3. Prostate gland – Diseases. 4. Afferent pathways – Diseases. I. George, N.J.R. (Nicholas James Robert), 1946– . II. Gosling, J.A. (John Arthur), 1939–
[DNLM: 1. Bladder Diseases – diagnosis. 2. Cystitis – diagnosis. 3. Prostatic Diseases – diagnosis. 4. Sensation. 5. Urethral Diseases – diagnosis. WJ 500 S478] RC919.S46 1985 616.6 85-26193

Softcover reprint of the hardcover 1st edition 1986

Filmset by Wilmaset, Birkenhead, Merseyside

2128/3916-543210

Foreword

The anticipation of seeing and having to manage patients suffering from sensory disorders of the urinary tract brings dismay and foreboding to the urologist. This stems from his experience of the time that these patients take up, both at the stage of initial interview and subsequently during numerous consultations over periods of months and years. This and the largely unsatisfactory response to various forms of therapy in the past are reason enough for this bold attempt to define with objectivity the notoriously subjective disorders of interstitial cystitis, urethral syndrome and prostatodynia.

In writing this book the principal aim of the authors has been to define these three entities concisely and to describe the investigational methods which are required to establish the diagnosis in each case. The importance of this cannot be overestimated since, when the label of one or other of these conditions is attached to a patient, further objective consideration of the case is endangered. The casual attribution of these sensory diagnoses to inappropriate cases is already on record as having dulled clinical awareness and led to oversight of progressive disease and its sometimes avoidable consequences.

In respect of interstitial cystitis there are several new observations of great interest which take us some way in the elucidation of the nature of this disease. The sections devoted to the urethral syndrome and prostatodynia show how much better the latter is defined as long as all of the recommended screening tests are performed. From this it is apparent that the urethral syndrome still requires more objective clinical and laboratory investigation than has so far been used to make this diagnosis.

To date the clinical management of patients with sensory disorders has relied heavily on an admixture of unsubstantiated observation, empirical drug therapy and personal whim. Good clinical trials of treatment have been few. It is to be hoped that the acceptance of precise urodynamic, microbiological and other definitive criteria will lead to a more disciplined investigative approach to diagnosis and more rational forms of treatment, such as are described in this volume. Hopefully, too, this will discourage the further influx of unscientific and irrational observation to the already large pool of unsatisfactory contributions which have served in the past only to confuse and discourage objective endeavour.

Manchester Professor N. J. Blacklock

Preface

"A Hole in the Air"

This lucid description of the sensory disorders, once advanced by Dr. Tage Hald in a moment of far-sighted wisdom, reflects perfectly the challenge offered to those who wish to understand the nature of sensory bladder and urethral dysfunction. These nebulous and poorly defined conditions have for years languished in various corners of the literature, brought to light only by the occasional monograph; difficulties of recognition and diagnosis ensure that comprehensive accounts are rarely to be found in the standard text of Urology and Gynaecology.

Sensation, abnormal or otherwise, cannot be other than a subjective experience which the physician must interpret as best as he is able. The exclusion of microbiological cause for disease requires painstaking and meticulous study of the lower urinary tract, often over an extended period of time, and the recognition and identification of urodynamic abnormality as a cause of symptoms will be no less demanding of the hard-pressed clinician. Thus the diagnosis of a sensory disorder is presently an exhaustive process of diagnosis by exclusion. From the complex mix of patients, symptoms and signs, each pathological entity must in turn be identified and eliminated until finally there remains a pool of patients in whom no cause can be found to account for their disease. These patients constitute the very substance of the "hole in the air"; the boundary is formed by those who have been identified and abstracted by due clinical process.

In the future specific techniques may be developed with which to diagnose such patients, and the availability of a group of highly screened cases will no doubt speed the introduction of appropriate tests to clinical practice. Until that time the Urologist, Microbiologist, Venereologist and Gynaecologist will need to rely on such specific descriptive accounts as are available, and hence this book brings together for the first time the historical, clinical, diagnostic and therapeutic aspects of the sensory dysfunctions. The combined approach allows a refreshingly clear view and reappraisal of those neglected patients who to date are unfortunate enough to consitute the subject matter of "the hole in the air".

June 1985 N. J. R. George

Contents

SECTION 2 INTERSTITIAL CYSTITIS

SECTION 3 THE URETHRAL SYNDROME

Contributors

R. J. Barnard, FRCS
Consultant Urological Surgeon, University Hospital of South Manchester, Manchester M20 8LR, England

P. J. C. Brooman, FRCS
Consultant Urological Surgeon, Stepping Hill Hospital, Stockport SK2 7JE, England

J. S. Dixon, BSc, PhD
Senior Lecturer in Histology, Department of Anatomy, University of Manchester, Medical School, Oxford Road, Manchester M13 9PT, England

C. A. C. Charlton, MS, FRCS
Consultant Urological Surgeon, Royal United Hospital, Bath BA1 3NG, England

N. J. R. George, FRCS
Lecturer and Senior Registrar in Urology, University Hospital of South Manchester, Manchester M20 8LR, England

T. Hald, MD, DMSc
Chief Urologist, Herlev Hospital, Copenhagen, Denmark

Marete Holm-Bentzen, MD
Research Associate in Urology, Herlev Hospital, Copenhagen, Denmark

P. King
Clinical Psychologist, Department of Psychology, University Hospital of South Manchester, Manchester M20 8LR, England

D. E. Osborn, MS, FRCS
Consultant Urological Surgeon, Leicester Royal Infirmary, Leicester, England

P. H. Powell, MD, FRCS
Consultant Urological Surgeon, Freeman Hospital, Newcastle upon Tyne, England

C. Reading
Principal Clinical Psychologist, Department of Psychology, University Hospital of South Manchester, Manchester M20 8LR, England

Shirley J. Richmond, MD
Senior Lecturer in Virology, Department of Bacteriology and Virology, University of Manchester, Medical School, Oxford Road, Manchester M13 9PT, England

Hilary Roberts
Research Psychologist, Department of Psychology, University Hospital of South Manchester, Manchester M20 8LR, England

Margaret Tasker, MB, ChB, MRCOG
Senior Registrar in Gynaecology, St. Mary's Hospital, Manchester M13 0JH, England

Section 1

Basic Considerations

Chapter 1

Introduction and Definitions

N. J. R. George

Difficulties in Definition

Until relatively recently the basic mechanisms which control the function of the human lower urinary tract were essentially unknown. However, the advent of sophisticated electromanometric techniques enabled considerable progress to be made in pressure and flow analyses within the bladder and urethra (Cardus et al. 1963). Attention was first directed towards motor abnormalities of the lower urinary tract, detrusor contraction waves being vividly recorded by increasingly sophisticated means. Thus scientific discussion commonly centred around the unstable bladder, obstructive voiding and urethral pressure profiles (Bates 1971; Turner-Warwick et al. 1973; Brown and Wickham 1969). Nevertheless, as information accumulated, it became evident that there were a number of disorders which, despite the presence of severe symptoms apparently originating from bladder or urethra, characteristically produced only minor changes on cystometry. These subtle changes were particularly difficult to interpret because of a lack of detailed control data.

The presence of symptoms emanating from the lower urinary tract combined with the lack of motor abnormalities on cystometric examination has led such patients to be designated as having a 'sensory' disorder of either bladder or urethra. This diagnosis to some extent begs the question, as there is no actual proof that the patient has a 'sensory' problem; the situation is more that the patient does *not* apparently have a motor disorder. This negative definition creates its own difficulties—there may in fact be no local abnormality or it may be that the urodynamic tests as employed are too insensitive to detect any subtle physiological changes that are taking place.

A similar problem of negative definition faces the clinician searching for evidence of lower urinary tract infection in these patients. Although symptoms of frequency and dysuria suggest the possibility of urinary infection, satisfactorily collected urine specimens frequently reveal a 'non-significant' level of bacterial growth. It is difficult in these circumstances for the clinician to interpret such reports, for if the organism is in fact responsible for the complex of symptoms then clearly a reappraisal of the definition of 'significance' is required (Mond et al. 1965; Brooks and Mauder 1972). On the other hand, if the report is taken as is implied, a search for other aetiological factors will be necessary (Charlton et al. 1973). In part this problem is related to the interpretation of indirect urine samples. The analysis of urine obtained directly from the bladder (for example by suprapubic aspiration) presents few difficulties for the microbiologist. During urethral voiding, however, the 'indirect' midstream collection is exposed to bacterial contamination, and judgement is then required as to whether the voided specimen of urine is truly representative of the urine present in the lower urinary tract.

Concise definitions of sensory disorders of the lower urinary tract vary according to local opinion. A number of specialities may be involved—urology, gynaecology or venereology—and opportunities rarely arise for these clinical specialists to meet and discuss common ground. Additionally, the populations served by these clinicians often differ significantly in terms of age, prevalence of disease, exposure to infectious agents, social behaviour and other epidemiological factors. For example, the patients presenting with urethral disorders to the Student Health Service of a University Campus will differ from those seen by a urologist at a District Hospital out-patient clinic. Although each speciality will naturally tend to concentrate on its own particular patients and patterns of disease, considerable benefit would be expected to derive from discussion with other inter-related and interested disciplines.

Finally it is generally agreed that many of the 'sensory' disorders are extremely difficult to treat with any degree of lasting success. It is clear that efforts to define those conditions of the lower urinary tract which are characterised as being sensory in nature will require rigorous attention to clinical detail, urodynamic definition and bacteriological methodology.

The Hypersensitive Disorders of Micturition

It has been noted that the construction of precise definitions of these disorders will be particularly difficult. This text refers almost entirely to *enhanced* sensation referrable to the lower urinary tract. Sensations experienced relating to the normal urinary tract are described on p. 7. States involving diminished sensation remain poorly understood and are not considered further in this book.

The description of a disorder as 'sensory' implies first and foremost that the symptoms are not related to active contraction of the detrusor. The conditions may be defined as having *an increase in perceived sensory stimulus from the bladder or urethra in the absence of urinary infection or detrusor contraction.* Thus the patient experiences sensation arising in the lower urinary tract which has not apparently resulted from either of these potential stimuli. This negative diagnosis cannot be reached without microbiological or urodynamic examination.

Before detailed consideration is given to each of these three definitive criteria (see Chap. 3) it is important first to describe sensation as experienced by normal persons (Chap. 2) and then to exclude two aspects of lower tract dysfunction which, though sensory in type, are not readily identified with the problematical clinical conditions described elsewhere in this text. These two aspects are the sensation associated with painful voiding and the sensory hypersensitivity that can occur in male patients with outflow tract obstruction (p. 17).

References

Bates CP (1971) Continence and incontinence: A clinical study of the dynamics of voiding and of the sphincter mechanisms. Ann R Coll Surg Engl 49:18–35

Brooks D, Mauder A (1972) Pathogenesis of the urethral syndrome in women and its diagnosis in general practice. Lancet II:893–899

Brown M, Wickham JEA (1969) The urethral pressure profile. Br J Urol 41:211–217

Cardus D, Quesada EM, Scott FB (1963) Studies on the dynamics of the bladder. J Urol 90:425–433

Charlton CAC, Cattell WR, Canti G, Grottick J, O'Grady FW (1973) The non urethral syndrome. In: Brumfitt W, Asscher AW (eds) Urinary tract infection. Oxford University Press, Oxford, pp 173–177

Mond NC, Percival A, Williams JD, Brumfitt W (1965) Presentation, diagnosis and treatment of urinary tract infections in general practice. Lancet I:514–516

Turner Warwick R, Whiteside GG, Arnold EP et al. (1973) A urodynamic view of prostatic obstruction and the results of prostatectomy. Br J Urol 45:631–645

Chapter 2

Normal Sensation of the Lower Urinary Tract

N.J.R. George and J.S. Dixon

Description of Normal Sensation

This chapter provides an account of normal bladder and urethral sensation and the anatomical pathways taken by sensory nerve impulses arising from the lower urinary tract. Description of the hypersensitive disorders is included in subsequent chapters.

Filling Phase

Following a void, the normal individual experiences no sensation from the lower urinary tract until the bladder has accumulated 200–300 ml of urine. At these values a vague sensation or 'tickle' may be experienced from an area which most people describe as being localised in the zone of the posterior urethra and this is the first conscious indication that the bladder is filling. This initial sensation, commonly referred to as the first desire to micturate (a rather inaccurate description as the feeling is usually slight and often waxes and wanes), eventually becomes persistent, thus persuading the person to seek a place to void. In these circumstances the *physiological bladder capacity* has been reached, its value being 400–550 ml of fluid. It is important to appreciate that even at this stage urethral or periurethral sensation may disappear from consciousness if some other pressing consideration intrudes. Only later does the desire to micturate return to disturb the individual's consciousness. This normal pattern is quite distinct from that seen in motor bladder disorders (bladder instability) where postponement of voiding is often impossible regardless of any other distractions that may be taking place.

If voiding is further postponed a second and separate sensation arises in addition to the persistent and by now almost painful periurethral discomfort. This sensation is manifest as a dull ache in the midline suprapubic region and is presumably related either to over-stretching of the bladder wall or to abnormal distension of the peritoneal covering of the bladder.

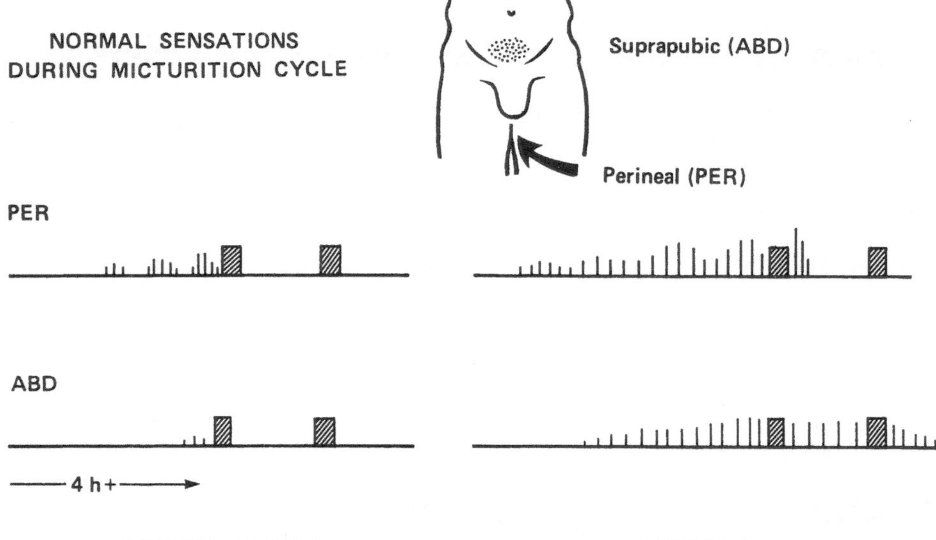

Fig. 2.1. Annotation for recording sensation during the micturition cycle. *Vertical strokes*, intensity of sensation. *Blocks*, start and finish of voiding. *PER*, posterior urethral or perineal sensation. *ABD*, suprapubic sensation. A record may be made for both normal and abnormal states (see text).

Voiding Phase

Micturition is usually sensation free although urethral distension and warmth can be detected (Nathan and Smith 1951). If voiding has been delayed there may be transient urethral discomfort at the commencement of the stream accompanied by a dull suprapubic ache, typically lasting a few minutes.

In taking a history from a patient it can be tedious to describe these sensations repeatedly in writing and a form of shorthand akin to cardiological records may be found to be convenient. Sensation is recorded along two lines which represent periurethral and suprapubic areas of sensation and relevant times may be noted if required (Fig. 2.1).

Anatomical and Physiological Considerations

Most investigators agree that whilst little is known of the detailed motor control of the normal lower urinary tract, even less is understood of the origin of sensory impulses from this region. As Mundy (1984) has pertinently observed, speculation and bias may commonly replace fact in accounts of the physiology of the bladder and urethra. In this chapter available data are summarised under the headings of sensory end organs, peripheral nerve pathways and central pathways within the cord. Connections at a higher level within and above the midbrain generally fall outside the terms of reference of this work.

Sensory End Organs

Anterior Urethra

The urothelial lining of the anterior urethra is sensitive to touch, thermal stimulation and pain (Nathan and Smith 1951). The ability of the normal person to witness these sensations is readily verified by perfusing the urethra with fluid at the appropriate temperature or slightly distending the urethra with an injection of lubricant gel.

Histologically an extensive plexus of nerve fibres has been demonstrated throughout the lamina propria of the human urethra in both males and females (Fig. 2.2a,b). These nerves are especially dense immediately beneath the epithelial lining of the urethra and are believed to subserve a sensory function. However, specialised sensory endings similar to those in the dermis of the skin have not been reported to occur in the wall of the urethra. Using electron microscopy such nerves are observed in close proximity to the basal aspect of the urethral epithelium. Many appear varicose and contain axonal vesicles which are of two morphologically distinct types (Fig. 2.2c). The majority have diameters of 40–60 nm and have a 'clear' interior, being referred to as agranular vesicles. The second type of vesicle is larger, with a diameter varying from 80 to 120 nm, and is characterised by the presence of a central dense granule.

Urethral Sphincter Zone

Passage of a urethral catheter in a patient is instructive as regards sensation emanating from the level of the external sphincter. Following the 'tactile'—but not painful—passage of the catheter along the distal urethra and (in the male patient) round the bulb, most patients describe a marked increase in sensation as the catheter passes through the level of the pelvic floor. The investigator has to exert additional force to advance the catheter at this point and the impression is that the muscles are relaxing to admit the tip of the catheter. The sensation is usually described as similar to that at the onset of micturition, but after 10 or 15 s it fades and the patient is then unaware of the catheter within the posterior urethra. The implication is that receptors which have responded to alteration of stretch adapt to the increased urethral diameter.

The terminology applied to the 'external urethral sphincter' requires clarification. In the past many authorities have referred to that part of the pelvic floor adjacent to the urethra, which is supplied by the pudendal nerve, as the 'external urethral sphincter' (Fletcher and Bradley 1978). In this text such striated muscle is described as being the *periurethral* muscle and the term external urethral sphincter is reserved for the anatomically distinct structure that is separated from the pelvic floor by a sleeve of connective tissue. The external urethral sphincter is thought to be mainly responsible for urinary continence and is supplied by branches of the pelvic nerve.

A plexus of subepithelial presumptive sensory nerve axons occurs at the level of the male external sphincter, similar to that described in the anterior urethra. However, it is interesting to note that specialised sensory endings of the type

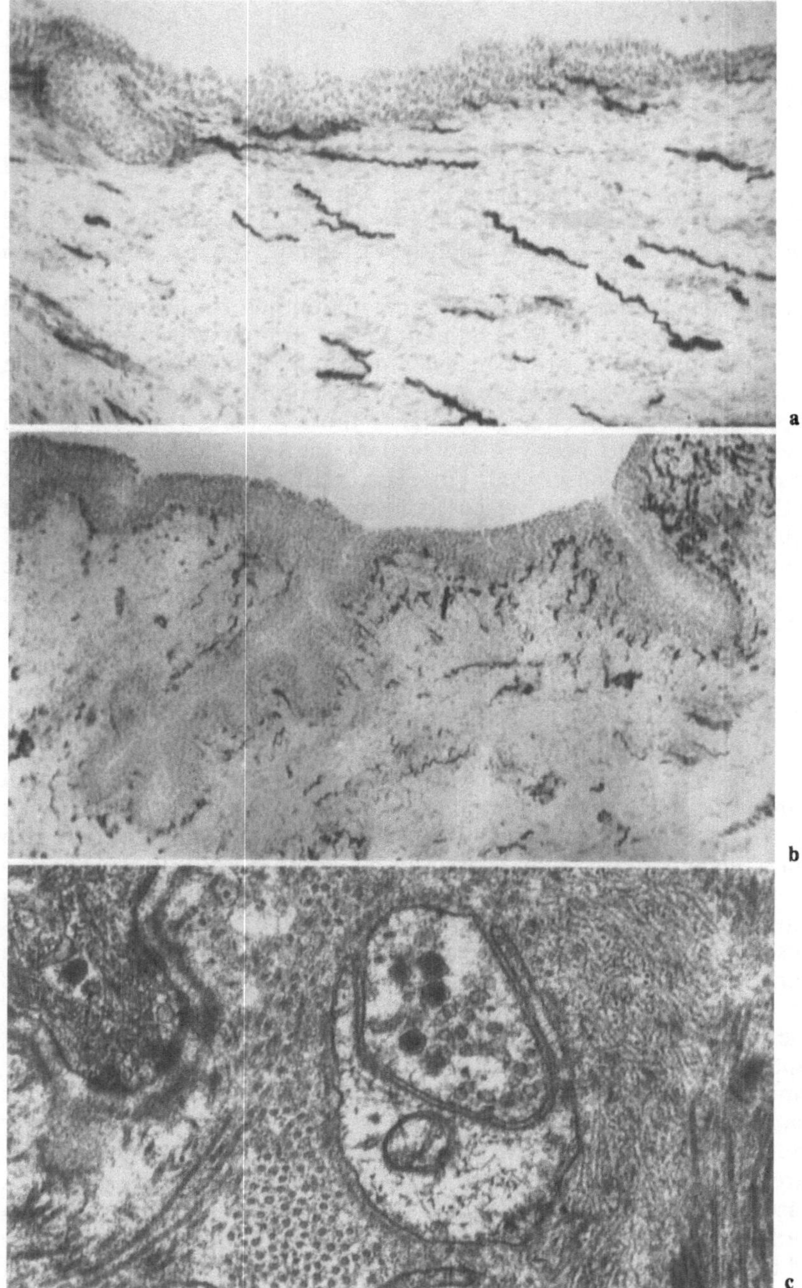

Fig. 2.2. a A plexus of nerve fibres is identified by an acetylcholinesterase technique beneath the epithelium of the male urethra. (× 250) **b** Acetylcholinesterase-positive nerve fibres form an extensive plexus in the lamina propria of the female urethra. (× 250) **c** Electron micrograph of a subepithelial axonal varicosity from the female urethra. The axon contains numerous small agranular vesicles and a few large granulated vesicles. (× 42 000)

found within striated muscle (i.e. muscle spindles) do not occur in the external urethral sphincter (Gosling et al. 1983). Muscle spindles do, however, occur within the periurethral striated muscle of the pelvic floor. No other specialised sensory endings have been observed within this region of the urethral wall.

Posterior Urethra, Trigone and Bladder Vault

Afferent activity from these areas is ultimately involved in the basic reflex control of micturition. The location of proprioceptive receptors which respond to changes in bladder wall tension or volume are not known at the present time, although their rate of discharge may be dependent upon the speed of bladder filling (Klevmark 1974). Stimuli affecting the trigone produce the classical symptom of strangury, pain referred along the urethra and a marked alteration of reflex activity (often experienced as severe frequency and urgency of micturition). It is occasionally observed that patients who have a calculus located within the terminal 2–3 cm of the ureter may also experience similar alterations in reflex activity. Sensation from inflamed mucosa within the bladder vault is usually described as a dull suprapubic ache. Whether this symptom represents involvement of visceral peritoneum or inflammation of the bladder wall alone is not known. Suction on a catheter in the bladder, which draws urothelium into a side hole, may also cause pain, particularly in patients with cystitis. Thermal sensation is probably not specifically distinguished by sensory receptors within the bladder (Nathan 1952).

At physiological volumes the bladder dome is not consciously appreciated, although overdistension may induce a dull suprapubic ache. This sensation may be transmitted by afferent endings in the peritoneal covering of the bladder. The possibility that the full bladder may, by gravitational means, influence proprioceptive receptors in the muscles of the pelvic floor cannot be discounted.

It is well known that a fine plexus of nerve fibres similar to those seen in the urethra occurs in the lamina propria of the bladder wall. These fibres present a characteristic appearance when viewed in the electron microscope (Fig. 2.3). Such nerves increase in density from the dome to the base of the bladder, being particularly numerous beneath the trigone and around the bladder neck. In the absence of any obvious affector site it is assumed that such nerves subserve a sensory function. It is interesting to note that recent immunofluorescence studies have demonstrated the presence of substance P in the subepithelial nerves of the human bladder, a substance that has been implicated in the transmission of sensory impulses (Alm et al. 1979).

Peripheral Nerve Pathways

Afferent impulses originating in the sensory nerve endings pass to the cord via the pudendal, pelvic and hypogastric nerves. By observation and experimentation the routes of impulses have become reasonably well established (Fig. 2.4).

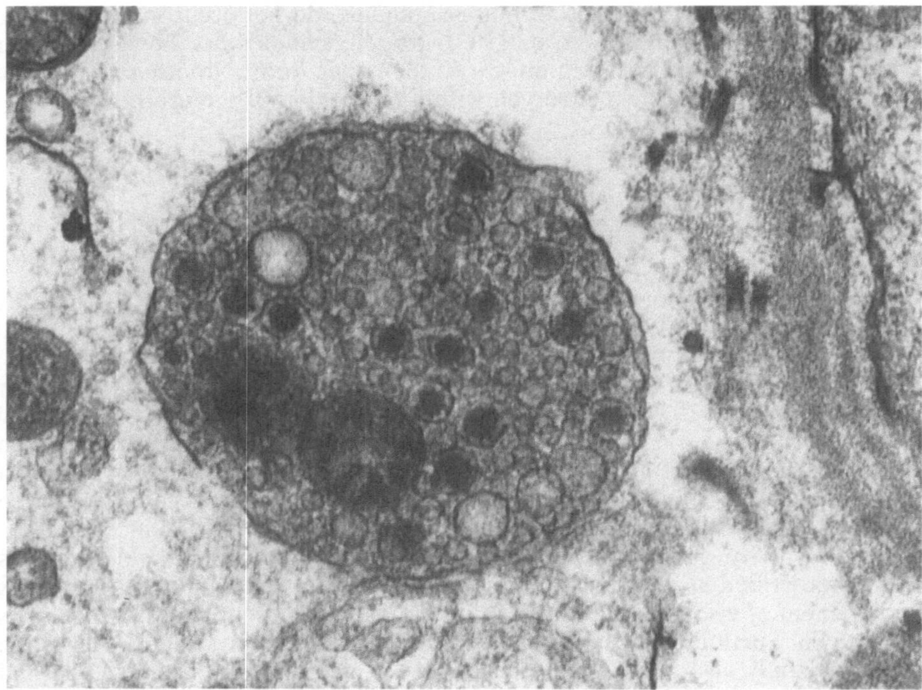

Fig. 2.3. Electron micrograph of a subepithelial nerve terminal from the trigone of the human urinary bladder. The nerve is completely devoid of a covering of neurilemmal cell and is packed with both small and large agranular vesicles together with numerous large granulated vesicles. (× 56 000)

Pudendal Nerve

The pudendal nerve transmits sensation from the skin of the genital area, the anal canal and urethral mucosa, and proprioceptive impulses from the periurethral striated sphincter muscle. It seems likely that the sensations described above, which are experienced as a catheter is passed into the bladder, are transmitted in this nerve as they are abolished by bilateral pudendal nerve block.

Pelvic Nerve

The afferent pathway of the micturition reflex is carried in the pelvic nerve (Learmonth 1931). The anatomical origin of the proprioceptive impulses together with those afferents concerned with bladder mucosal pain and lower ureteric pain which also pass in the pelvic nerve remains uncertain.

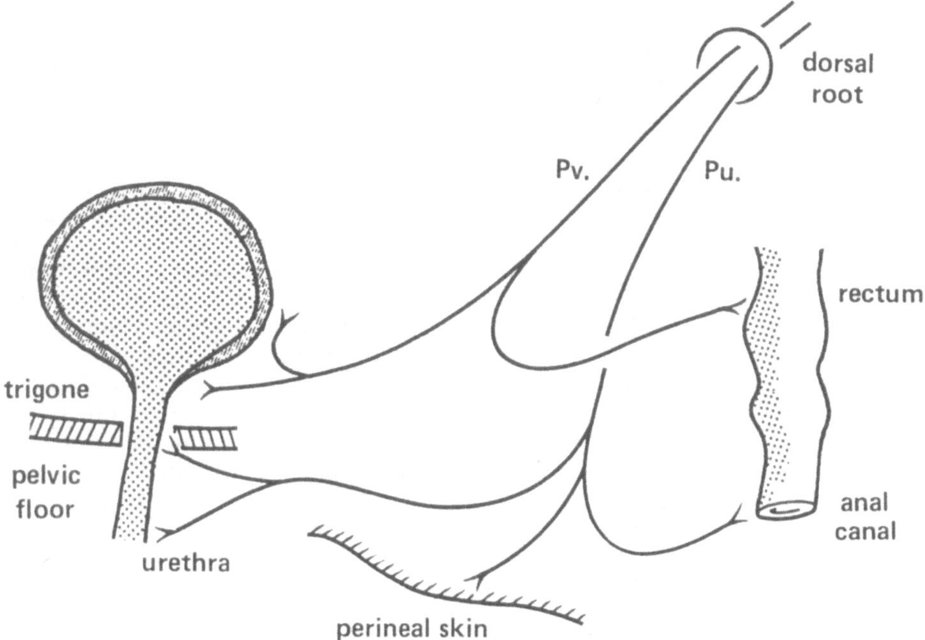

Fig. 2.4. Afferent pathways from caudal structures. *Pv*, pelvic nerve: *Pu*, pudendal nerve.

Hypogastric Nerve

The part played by the hypogastric nerve in relaying sensation from the lower urinary tract is unknown. No alteration in bladder or urethral sensation occurs after presacral neurectomy (Learmonth 1931), though some sensation of fullness has occasionally been noted to be preserved after lower spinal injury (Head and Riddoch 1917).

Relative Importance of Nerve Pathways in the Physiology of Micturition

Afferent activity passing by either somatic or autonomic pathways may play a part in the physiology of micturition. Stimulation of the S1 or S2 dermatome by pain or cold fluids commonly promotes voiding, especially in children (personal observation.) Curiously, painful pinching of perianal skin did not affect detrusor contraction waves in the experiments of Kock and Pompeius (1963) whilst detrusor instability was abolished by penile squeeze in 17 of 20 patients studied by Kondo et al. (1982). The passage of a urethral catheter through the periurethral sphincter muscle zone produces a marked, though short-lived, desire to void in normal persons (Nathan and Smith 1951).

Conversely, a normal person will find that it is impossible to state at any particular time whether his bladder is empty or half-full. Recording from the pelvic nerve of cats Iggo (1955) was able to detect activity which disappeared when the bladder relaxed. Such ‘subconscious’ centripetal impulses may additionally be modified by various factors. Annis (1962) reported an alteration of the micturition reflex which was related to abnormal bladder mucosal sensibility and these findings were confirmed by Sabetian (1965). Recently the application of lignocaine to the trigonal area has been found to increase bladder capacity and alter the character of the cystometrogram during cystometry (George 1978; Higson et al. 1979; Reuther et al. 1983). These observations, taken together, support the contention that sensory impulses arising from the bladder and posterior urethra do not reach consciousness, at least in the early stages of bladder filling.

The central issue concerns the source and route taken by afferent information that is essential for normal micturition; that is, information without which the fundamental events of the micturition reflex will not take place. Clinical and radiological studies on patients without neurological abnormalities have shown that, following bilateral pudendal nerve block, micturition is normal and can be initiated at will (Emmett et al. 1948; Lapides et al. 1955; Raz and Smith 1976). In contradistinction, fibres carried in the pelvic nerve are presumed by a process of exclusion to be of critical importance, as bilateral section of these nerves results in severe functional abnormalities of both storing and voiding phases of the micturition cycle (Learmonth 1931; for review see Kuru 1965). From these studies it may be concluded that afferent impulses passing in the pudendal nerve are not *essential* for normal reflex micturition (Table 2.1).

Table 2.1. Origin, course and destination of sensory impulses from caudal structures

	To posterior column	To anterolateral column
From pudendal nerve (non-essential)	Exteroception – urethral mucosa – anal canal Proprioception – peri-urethral sphincter	Pain, Temperature } urethral mucosa
From pelvic nerve (essential)		Pressure/volume sensors (afferent arm micturition reflex) Pain – bladder mucosa – lower ureters Distension – rectum

Sensory Innervation from Other Organs

Stimuli from other organs may affect urogenital function. An overdistended rectum is frequently associated, especially in the elderly, with an inability to empty the bladder completely. Mechanical obstruction of the bladder outlet is not always present in these circumstances and it is possible that altered afferent activity from such an overdistended viscus might adversely affect reflex activity concerned with the bladder and urethra. Rectal distension was shown to affect pelvic floor activity by Porter (1962), whilst anal distension inhibited detrusor contraction in the normal subjects investigated by Kock and Pompeius (1963).

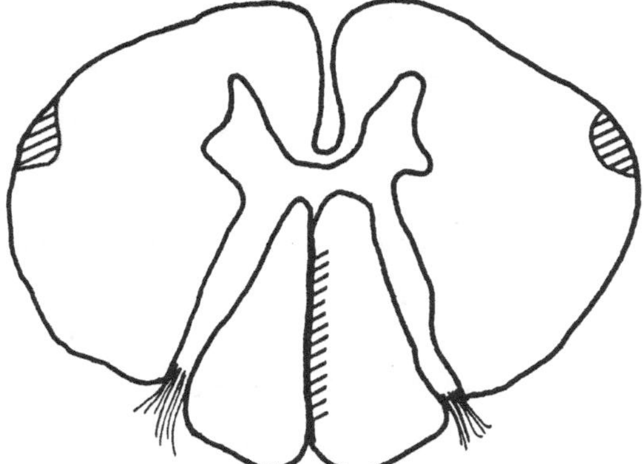

Fig. 2.5. Transverse section of spinal cord at midthoracic level. Lateral funiculus: vesical proprioception; pain from urethra and lower end of ureter; temperature from urethra. Posterior columns: touch, pressure and tension from urethra. (After Nathan and Smith 1951)

Spinal Pathways

By careful observation of patients undergoing anterolateral cordotomy, Nathan and Smith (1951) have deduced that impulses concerned with the sensation of bladder fullness (afferent limb of micturition reflex), pain from bladder and urethral mucosa, and temperature from the urethra, pass within the spinothalamic tracts. Impulses concerned with urethral proprioception and touch ascend via the dorsal columns (Fig. 2.5).

The fundamental reflex arc concerning micturition has its nuclei in the brainstem at the intercollicular level—the pontine micturition centre. Afferent neurones that have ascended in the lateral funiculus synapse at this level but those axons concerned with urethral touch and proprioception terminate in the region of the gracile nuclei.

References

Alm P, Alumets K, Ek A, Sundler F (1979) Peptidergic (VIP) nerves in the human urinary tract Proc. Ninth Int Cont Soc Meeting, Rome, p 147

Annis D (1962) Evidence concerning function of mucosa in reflex act of micturition. Ann R Coll Surg Engl 31:23–45

Emmett JL, Daut RV, Dunn JH (1948) Role of the external urethral sphincter in the normal bladder and cord bladder. J Urol 59:439–454

Fletcher TF, Bradley WE (1978) Neuroanatomy of the bladder-urethra. J Urol 119: 153–160

George NJR (1978) Influence of lignocaine on bladder instability. Paper presented at VIIIth meeting of the International Continence Society. Manchester

Gosling JA, Dixon JS, Humperson JR (1983) Functional anatomy of the urinary tract. Churchill Livingstone, London

Head H, Riddoch G (1917) The automatic bladder, excessive sweating and some other reflex conditions in gross injuries of the spinal cord. Brain 40:188–263

Higson RH, Smith JC, Hills W (1979) Intravesical lignocaine and detrusor instability. Br J Urol 51: 500–503

Iggo A (1955) Tension receptors in the stomach and urinary bladder. J Physiol (Lond) 128:593

Klevmark B (1974) Motility of the urinary bladder in cats during filling at physiological rates. I. Intravesical pressure patterns studied by a new method of cystometry. Acta Physiol Scand 90:565–577

Kock NG, Pompeius R (1963) Inhibition of vesical motor activity induced by anal stimulation. Acta Chir Scand 126:224–250

Kondo A, Otari T, Takita T (1982) Suppression of bladder instability by penile squeeze. Br J Urol 54: 360–362

Kuru M (1965) Nervous control of micturition. Physiol Rev 45:425–494

Lapides J, Gray HO, Rawling JC (1955) Function of striated muscles in control of urination. (1) Effect of pudendal block. Surg Forum 6:611

Learmonth JR (1931) A contribution to the neurophysiology of the urinary bladder in man. Brain 54: 147–176

Mundy AR (1984) Clinical physiology of the bladder, urethra and pelvic floor. In: Mundy AR, Stephenson TP, Wein AJ (eds) Urodynamics, principles, practice and application. Churchill-Livingstone, Edinburgh, pp 14–15

Nathan PW (1952) Thermal sensation in the bladder. J Neurol Neurosurg Psychiatry 15:150–151

Nathan PW, Smith MC (1951) The centripetal pathway from the bladder and urethra within the spinal cord. J Neurol Neurosurg Psychiatry 14: 262–280

Porter NH (1962) A physiological study of the pelvic floor in rectal prolapse. Ann R Coll Surg Engl 31: 379–404

Raz S, Smith RB (1976) External sphincter spasticity syndrome in female patients. J Urol 115: 443–446

Reuther K, Aagaard J, Sander Jensen K (1983) Lignocaine test and detrusor instability. Br J Urol 55:493–494

Sabetian M (1965) The role of the vesical mucosa in reflex micturition. Br J Urol 37: 417–423

Chapter 3

Diagnostic Criteria of the Hypersensitive Disorders

N.J.R. George

Introduction

The hypersensitive disorders are recognised by an abnormal increase in perceived sensation from the lower urinary tract in the absence of bacteriological infection or detrusor contraction (p. 4). A detailed examination of each of these three criteria allows for clarity of clinical definition which in turn leads to a basis for classification of the sensory disorders. Firstly, however, it is necessary to describe two forms of sensation which, although abnormal, are not commonly associated with the clinical conditions described in later sections of this book.

Painful Voiding

The definition of a hypersensitive disorder applies in the main to the filling phase of the micturition cycle; it is during these hours that the patient's symptoms are at their worst. It has to be considered, however, that abnormal sensation may also occur during voiding and indeed micturition may occasionally be uncomfortable in those patients with the urethral syndrome or prostatodynia, probably due to some transient spasm or poor relaxation at sphincter level (Kaplan et al. 1980). As the degree of spasm increases, voiding will inevitably become increasingly painful, and to this extent some sensory disorders may be said to be a cause of dysuria. However, for clarity of definition abnormal sensation occurring during voiding (when a detrusor contraction is usually taking place) is probably best regarded as *not* being of critical importance in definitive accounts of the sensory disorders. It is not disputed that painful voiding occasionally occurs in patients with sensory disorders and that such symptoms are of clinical concern; no doubt such terms as the 'frequency dysuria syndrome' will continue in common clinical usage. The crucial factors, however, concerned with aetiology and diagnosis and upon which the sensory definitions are based are to be found during periods when voiding is not taking place.

Bladder Hypersensitivity and Outflow Tract Obstruction

Symptoms of lower urinary tract dysfunction related to bladder hypersensitivity have been described in patients with outflow tract obstruction secondary to prostatic hypertrophy (Abrams et al. 1979). Cystometric examination in these patients demonstrates stable bladders but an early first desire to micturate, leading to significantly reduced capacity at the termination of filling. Hypersensitivity has been defined by Abrams as occurring when functional bladder capacity is limited by either urethral or suprapubic discomfort to less than 250 ml (Abrams et al. 1981).

A detailed history obtained from an older man with cystometrically proven bladder hypersensitivity usually reveals that the desire to micturate is identified as a sensation originating from the normal posterior urethral zone; suprapubic discomfort is not a common complaint unless for any reason the bladder has become over-distended. Following micturition all sensation in the lower urinary tract usually disappears until the first desire to micturate returns. Hence patients with hypersensitivity related to outflow tract obstruction may be considered to have a mild form of sensory disturbance when comparison is made with the patient whose urethral discomfort commonly persists throughout the micturition cycle.

It might be postulated that the hypersensitivity associated with benign prostatic hypertrophy is related to local distortion factors occurring as a result of adenomatous growth at the base of the bladder. Some support for this theory is provided by the observation that local anaesthetics applied to the trigone and posterior urethral zone increase bladder capacity and residual urine during cystometric tests (George 1978; Higson et al. 1979). Whatever the aetiology of this type of hypersensitivity, however, the disorder stands apart from other conditions described in this text by virtue of the symptomatic resolution and cystometric improvement that occurs following routine resection of the prostate gland. It would seem reasonable to conclude that the mechanisms responsible for the hypersensitive state in the older man with prostatic hypertrophy must differ significantly from those involved in the prostatodynia symptom complex seen in younger men.

Sensation in the Hypersensitive Disorders

Abnormal sensation may be experienced in both urethral and suprapubic areas.

Urethral Sensation

Taking a history in the detail described on p. 7 is essential if one is to distinguish the various sensory disorders from each other, and a frequency and volume chart (see below, p. 35) will be an invaluable aid in this procedure. Such enquiries will

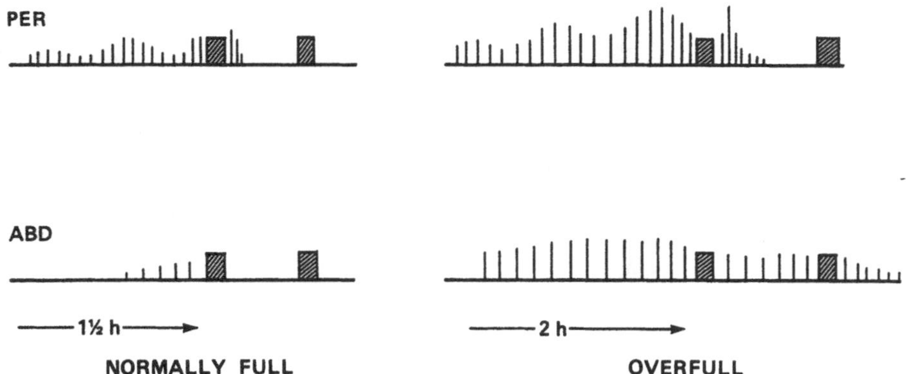

Fig. 3.1. Annotation in urethral hypersensitivity disorders. Persistent urethral 'niggle' and suprapubic ache if undue delay in micturition. Compare time scale with Fig. 2.1.

usually clearly distinguish those sensory disorders in which the abnormality is apparently located primarily in the urethra from those where the bladder appears to be the site of discomfort. The 'urethral syndrome' and 'prostatodynia' are typified by urethral discomfort which, in severe cases, persists throughout the filling and voiding cycle. However, it is important to note that the patient is only inconvenienced by the sensation and does not *have* to micturate—indeed many patients try to 'face it out' in an attempt to reduce their urinary frequency. This sensation is perhaps better described as sensory *irritation*, and should be distinguished from motor *urgency*, in which the patient has to void in order to avoid leakage of urine. Generally, when sensory patients are asked if they consider that they might wet themselves, they appear astonished as the possibility will not previously have occurred to them. If these patients delay micturition, in addition to the severe local urethral discomfort, bladder cramps may become marked, even when bladder volumes are small (Fig. 3.1).

Bladder Sensation

In those disorders where the abnormality apparently resides in the bladder (interstitial cystitis, post-radiation fibrosis, tuberculosis etc.) it is the dull suprapubic ache which is the patient's main complaint. The patient interprets this ache as being continuously 'over-full' and this sensation is thus identified as the signal to void. A urethral component can in fact, on careful enquiry, be distinguished, although this fails to predominate before the suprapubic discomfort dictates that voiding will occur. Figure 3.2 illustrates this form of sensory disorder.

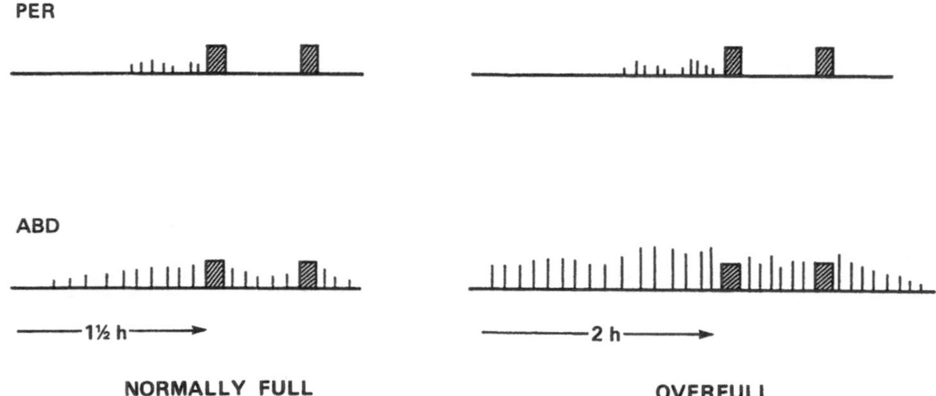

Fig. 3.2. Annotation in bladder 'vault' hypersensitivity. Urethral sensation is present but the driving desire for micturition is suprapubic in origin and this discomfort settles only slowly after voiding is completed.

The Psychological Perception of Abnormal Sensation

It will be appreciated that the lower urinary and genital tracts are psychologically 'sensitive' zones, and that perceived sensation may be enhanced if the patient concentrates unduly on the area in question. Hence, during urodynamic testing, the attention of the patient is distracted in an effort to avoid over-reaction to stimuli from the bladder or urethra.

Extraneous thoughts or stimuli from other areas may affect sensory awareness, for example, the idea of washing up dishes or the sound of running water. Nathan and Smith (1951) described a neurological patient who, despite having no sensation from her bladder, experienced the desire to micturate on seeing or hearing the sound of bedpans in the hospital ward. Such stimuli seem likely to act by modulating the activity of central reflex arcs rather than by enhancing sensory impulses from the periphery.

Given the subjectivity of 'perceived' sensation, it is possible that a neurologically normal patient may feel that sensory stimuli arising from the urinary tract are excessive, though both bladder and urethra are physiologically and bacteriologically normal. It may be that such patients have heightened awareness of stimuli (Fig. 3.3) and over-react to normal levels of afferent activity, much as do those who become anxious of their heart rate or the occurrence of occasional extrasystolic beats. Psychological aspects of lower urinary tract disorders have been studied by a number of workers (Rees and Farhoumand 1977; Carson et al. 1980; Keltikangas-Järvinen et al. 1981) and are also considered in the relevant sections of this book.

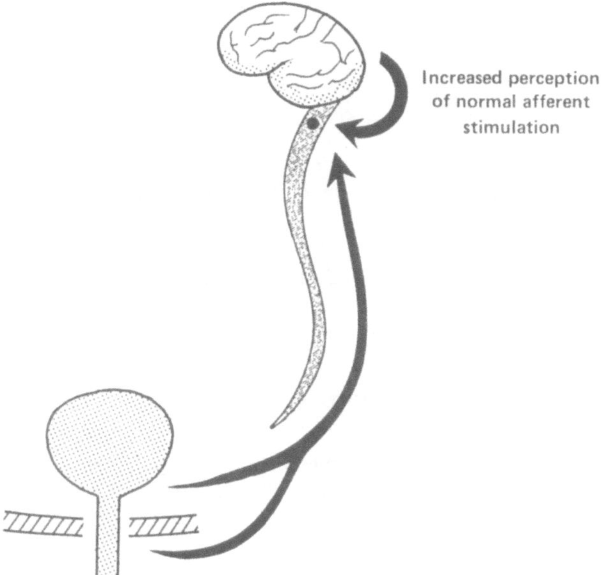

Fig. 3.3. The perception of sensation may be enhanced although normal afferent activity is arising from the lower urinary tract; such 'psychogenic' mechanisms may feed back to caudal structures via motor pathways leading to (for example) abnormal states of tension in pelvic floor muscles. This abnormality in turn may promote increased afferent activity and so on (see also Fig. 18.2, p. 166).

Classification of the Hypersensitive Disorders by the Origin of Abnormal Sensation

The forms of abnormal sensation described above provide a satisfactory means of classifying the hypersensitive disorders of the lower urinary tract.

Disorders Related to Enhanced Urethral Sensation

The importance of diagnosing organic disease (for example, urethral caruncle, genital herpes or tumour) by routine clinical process cannot be over-emphasised. Bacteriological considerations and the classification based thereon are described in detail on p. 24. Enhanced urethral sensation that is apparently unrelated to pathological change may occur in patients of either sex and these disorders are fully described in the sections beginning on pp. 79 and 123.

Disorders Related to Enhanced Bladder Sensation

Sensations from the bladder are referred to the suprapubic region and may be induced by conditions in which there is a physical limitation of bladder capacity. As with the urethral disorders it is important first to identify and exclude those patients with extrinsic or intrinsic bladder wall disease.

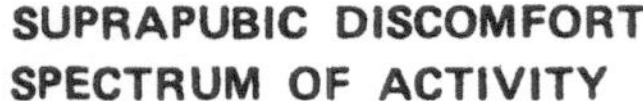

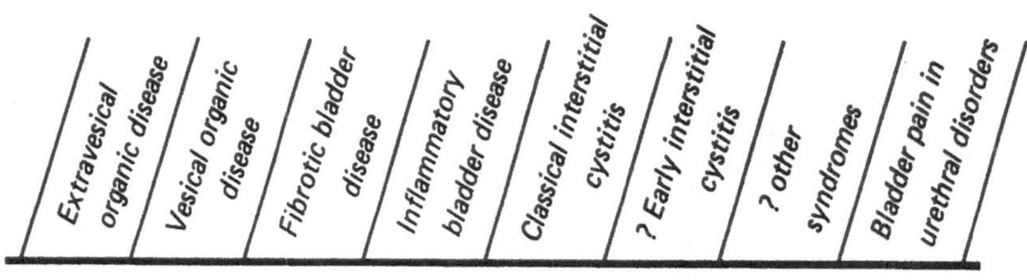

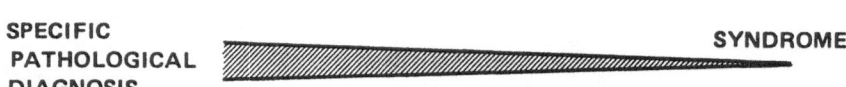

SPECIFIC PATHOLOGICAL DIAGNOSIS

SYNDROME

Fig. 3.4. The spectrum of disorders which may present with suprapubic discomfort. *Left*, specific pathological diagnoses blend, *right*, into poorly understood suprapubic 'syndromes' for which at present no explanation can be found.

The aetiology of the symptom complexes which arise from the bladder may be viewed along a graduated scale, the horizontal axis referring to histological findings on bladder biopsy (Fig. 3.4). To the left, diagnosis may be made in conjunction with other clinical findings of a specific pathological disorder; for example, fibrosis due to radiation, tuberculosis, carcinoma or other causes. Right shift passes through 'classical' interstitial cystitis, which is described in its most unequivocal form on p. 49. On further shift to the right, the equivocal case of interstitial cystitis blends into the suprapubic discomfort felt, for example, in some cases of the urethral syndrome in which bacteriological abnormality is absent.

Appreciation of the suprapubic spectrum of sensory abnormalities is important in that particular symptoms may not be so disease-specific as once thought. The appearance, for example, of haemorrhagic spots at the second cystoscopic filling of the bladder may be noted in some patients with symptom complexes which would not otherwise be recognised as being typical of interstitial cystitis. The diagnostic criteria of the suprapubic symptom complexes are presently unresolved and the clinician is best advised to be aware of the range of possibilities and await definition of the various disorders by new diagnostic techniques.

Bacteriological Considerations in the Diagnosis of the Hypersensitive Disorders

Consideration of the role of infection in the pathogenesis of sensory disorders of the lower urinary tract requires not only a working knowledge of the possible microbes involved, but also an appreciation of the problems concerned in the estimation and definition of bacteriological 'significance' that may be applied to these conditions. These problems can be particularly well illustrated by a study of the voided urine of female patients.

Bacteriological Significance

The quantitative estimation of organisms within any particular fluid or secretion will be an essential prerequisite for the formation of guidelines as to what numbers of those organisms constitute a significant clinical infection. Taking the example of urine from patients with pyelonephritis, it has been proposed that organisms in a concentration of greater than 10^5 per ml obtained from midstream urine imply the presence of significant infection (Kass 1955; Kass and Finland 1956). This guideline has frequently been followed not only for patients with upper tract infection but also for patients with suspected lower urinary tract disease, though the modifying effect of factors such as excessive fluid ingestion or antibiotic therapy has been well recognised for many years.

There is, however, no evidence that the criteria for renal infection should apply to the urinary tract as a whole. Stamm and co-workers (1982), studying female patients with frequency and acute dysuria (painful voiding) attending a University Student clinic, determined that a bacterial concentration of greater than 10^2 per ml in midstream urine was the diagnostic test which resulted in 'optimal sensitivity and specificity for purpose of management'. Only 51% of symptomatic patients whose bladder urine contained coliform organisms recovered by the suprapubic route were correctly diagnosed by applying traditional 'Kass criteria' to midstream urine. Similar observations were reported in a study of urban general practice patients in which only 45% had bacteriuria in concentrations of greater than 10^5 per ml. The importance of lesser concentrations of organisms was, however, emphasised by the presence of pyuria in half of the patients with 'non-significant' infection (Mond et al. 1965).

Bacterial counts of less than 10^2 per ml may rarely be found within the bladder urine of normal persons. Under certain circumstances, such as dehydration and voiding abstinence for several hours (i.e. overnight), organisms may be cultured in low concentration from suprapubic aspirates. Reasonable hydration and a normal voiding interval might be expected to prevent this ascent of microbes into bladder urine and under these conditions such urine should remain sterile.

On occasion the occurrence of coliforms in low concentration together with other isolates is treated as evidence of specimen contamination by a reporting laboratory. However, non-coliform isolates—chiefly *Staphylococcus saprophyticus*, *Staph. aureus* and enterococci—were detected by Stamm et al. (1982) in 26 of 89 symptomatic female patients, and these workers argued that urine yielding such mixed cultures and pyuria should not automatically be regarded as contaminated (Stamm 1984).

Thus the clinician cannot be offered rigid guidelines by which to pronounce bacteriological judgement on the midstream urine of his patients. The significance or otherwise of any microbiological observation will depend as much on the characteristics of the study population and the prevalence of disease as on the techniques of sampling, the chance of specimen contamination and specific laboratory methodology. Under these complex circumstances it is clear that only close cooperation between the interested parties is likely to result in a real advance in practical patient management.

Pyuria

The observation of large numbers of polymorphonuclear leucocytes together with numerous organisms in midstream urine does not constitute a diagnostic problem for either the clinician or the microbiologist. When, however, leucocytes occur in the presence of few organisms or in sterile urine, a more critical bacteriological assessment will generally be required in order to make a diagnosis. Further tests might include the study of aspirated bladder urine, as well as the culture of urethral, introital and cervical swabs, in an effort to determine the precise origin of the infection. Using such techniques evidence of recent infection with *Chlamydia trachomatis* was obtained in 10 of 16 patients with sterile pyuria, though no cause could be found for the pyuria in the remaining six patients (Stamm et al. 1980).

Classification of the Hypersensitive Disorders by Means of Bacteriological Criteria

The bacteriological criteria described allow a further means whereby the sensory disorders may be classified and this will particularly apply to those conditions in which the urethral zone is apparently the prime site of discomfort.

Specific Pathogenesis and Syndromes

One obstacle to continued progress in the understanding of sensory disorders is the lack of a rigidly defined framework of terminology to which urologists, gynaecologists, venereologists, bacteriologists and other workers can strictly adhere. The concept of a quantitative relationship between organisms and white cells in any physiological fluid enables these problems of terminology to be illustrated (Fig. 3.5). On the left of the scale there is little diagnostic difficulty in recognising that the patients have symptoms due to *acute bacterial inflammation*. As the quantitative counts decrease the pathogenesis becomes less certain until the reason for the symptoms in the patient with neither organisms nor white cells cannot presently be explained at all. These patients are therefore referred to as having a 'syndrome', the term implying a symptomatic description (e.g. frequency, dysuria) of a condition of unknown aetiology. These 'syndromes' are often described by different authors under different headings; for example, prostatodynia, pelvic floor myalgia, prostatosis, etc. in the male patient (Segura et al. 1979) (see p. 139).

The uncertainty therefore rests on where the line is drawn by the clinician between specific pathogenesis and descriptive 'syndrome'. Hence it might be a valid question to ask—assuming the criteria for detrusor contraction are

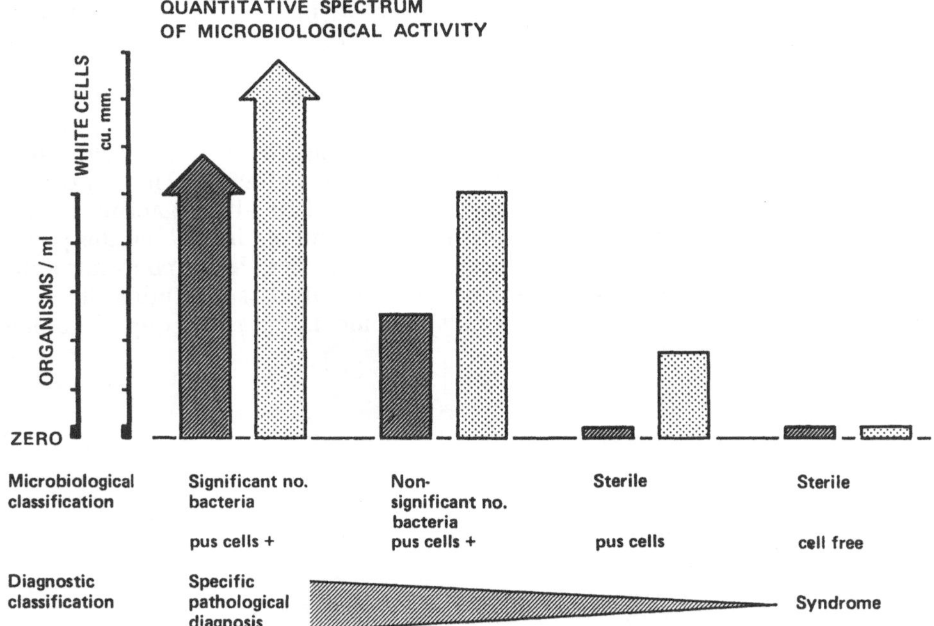

Fig. 3.5. The spectrum of microbiological activity. *Hatched columns*, bacteria per ml. *Shaded columns*, polymorphonuclear cells per mm^3. This form of analysis may be usefully employed in a number of situations. To the *left* large numbers of organisms and white cells imply significant bacterial infection. Right shift passes through conditions in which lesser numbers of organisms and white cells lead to interpretive difficulties. The symptoms in conditions on the *right* cannot be explained on a microbiological basis when conventional culture techniques are applied.

fulfilled—why patients with 'significant' infection should be excluded from having a 'sensory' disorder; clearly bacterial cystitis is painful. It would, however, seem reasonable to concentrate on that area of the spectrum where aetiological factors are in doubt and leave aside recognised disease. If necessary one can state for completeness' sake that a patient has a 'sensory disorder due to acute bacterial cystitis' or 'due to acute inflammatory prostatitis'.

Specific Problems Concerning the Terminology of the Symptom Complex Arising from the Urethral Zone

Female Patients. Few clinical conditions can have been assigned a greater number of diverse definitions than have been applied to the condition of the 'urethral syndrome' (Lancet 1982). It seems reasonable to propose that symptomatic patients without cells or organisms in midstream or bladder urine should constitute the true nucleus of the disorder. Patients with sterile pyuria may also be included under this heading although some patients will possess a specific abnormality on careful investigation (Stamm et al. 1980). Patients with a 'non-significant' bacteruria of 10^2–10^5 organisms per ml in midstream urine do not warrant the title of 'urethral syndrome' (Fig. 3.6).

These problems of terminology are very well illustrated by a recent study entitled the 'acute urethral syndrome' (Stamm et al. 1980). These workers initially included patients with frequency, dysuria and 10^2–10^5 organisms per ml in midstream urine within the spectrum of the 'urethral syndrome' but this paper and later work from the same centre concluded that these lesser concentrations of organisms were indeed of significance, thus effectively substituting the term 'unrecognised cystitis' for 'acute urethral syndrome' in this sub-group of women (Stamm et al. 1980, 1982).

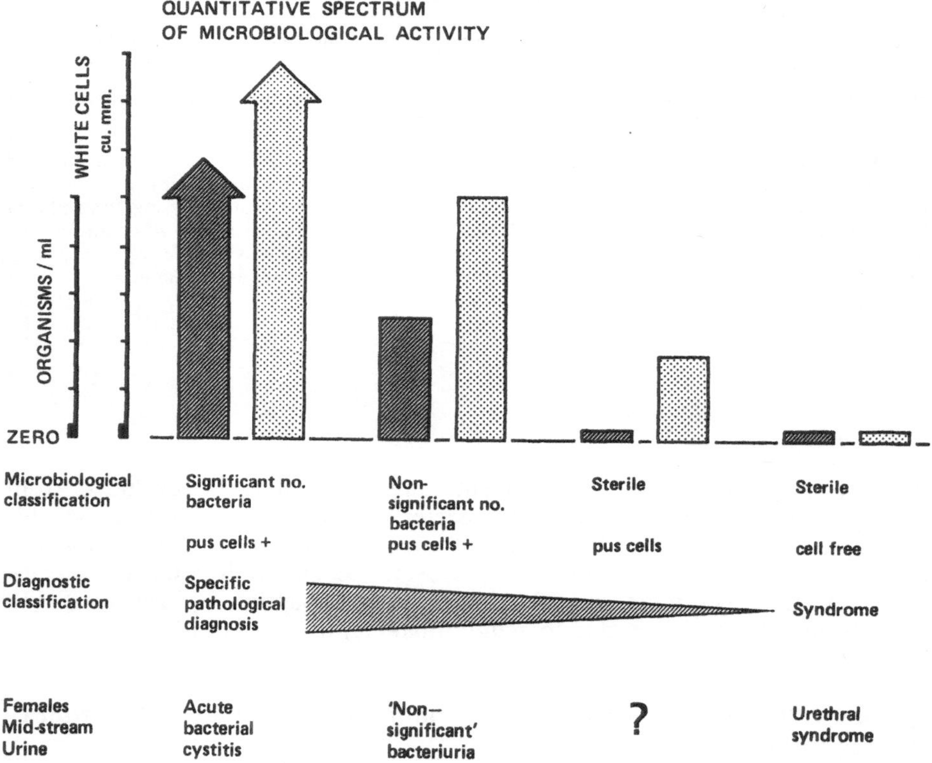

Fig. 3.6. The spectrum of microbiological activity applied to the findings within midstream (VB2) urine of female patients. Many authorities quote 'non-significant' levels of bacteriuria as concentrations less than 10^5 organisms per ml (Mond et al. 1965) though this is questioned by other workers (Brooks and Mauder 1972; Stamm et al. 1980, see text). Some patients with sterile pyuria may be included in the urethral syndrome but more critical microbiological assessment will identify a specific pathogen in a number of these cases.

Male Patients. Due to the work of Drach and associates (1978) the term 'prostatodynia' has been introduced to define a symptomatic group of male patients with cell-free sterile expressed prostatic secretion. Patients without evidence of bacteria in secretion which contains significant numbers of leucocytes are classified as having a 'non-bacterial' prostatitis, though changes in pH may provide some evidence of previous bacterial infection. Furthermore, a critical microbiological assessment of these cases may, as in female patients, imply the presence of a specific pathogen within the prostatic secretion (i.e. *Chlamydia trachomatis*, see Chap. 15 and Fig. 3.7).

The similarity between these two disorders will not have escaped the notice of the informed clinician, and it is true to say that those who best understand the picture of prostatodynia recognise most clearly the exact form of the urethral syndrome.

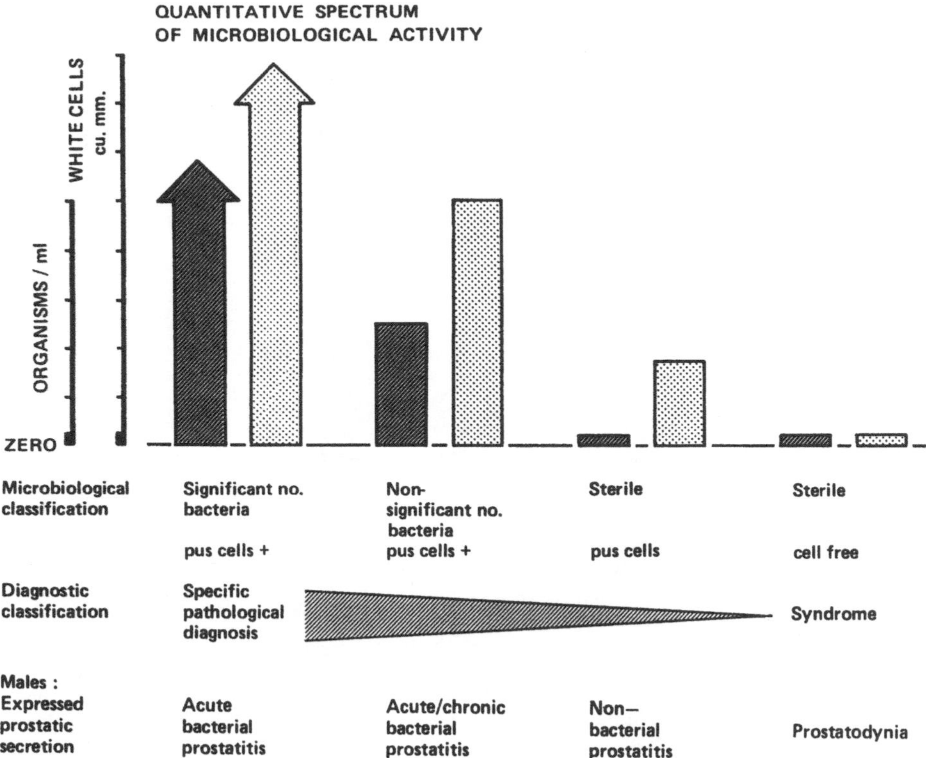

Fig. 3.7. The spectrum of microbiological activity applied to findings in expressed prostatic secretion. The classification of Drach et al. (1978) is satisfactory although bacteriological isolation rates in prostatitis are characteristically low and the distinction between acute and chronic prostatitis is generally made on clinical grounds rather than by identification of specific numbers of colony counts per ml. As with the spectrum in female patients, more critical evaluation of patients with non-bacterial prostatitis may identify a pathogen in a number of cases.

The Hypersensitive Disorders and Detrusor Contraction

The hypersensitive disorders show an insignificant detrusor pressure rise during bladder filling which is defined as being *less* than 15 cm H_2O at capacity (Fig. 3.8). The absence of detrusor contraction waves is essential for the diagnosis of a sensory disorder.

In conjunction with this minimal pressure rise, patients with sensory disorders often possess a reduced physiological bladder capacity. This reduction may be expressed clinically as an increase in the frequency of micturition. The sensation associated with the desire to void, however, is often enhanced and it is the combination of these factors—minimal pressure rise, a reduced conscious bladder capacity and enhanced sensation—that characterises the urodynamic findings during the filling phase in these patients.

Conclusion

The hypersensitive disorders of the lower urinary tract are defined in terms of symptoms which are experienced in the absence of either infection or detrusor contraction. These criteria may be considered to be imprecise when comparison

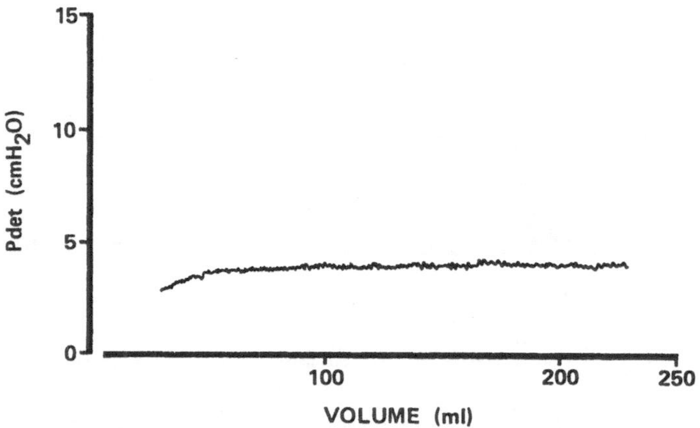

Fig. 3.8. Hypersensitive inflow cystometrogram. Minimal pressure rise during filling, the patient experiencing a 'normal' desire to void at 225 ml. The cystometrogram is a poor measure of the hypersensitive disorders as it does not record the patient's main complaint—abnormal sensation. Thus the distinction between a 'normal' and 'hypersensitive' inflow cystometrogram remains difficult and these two forms will meet at some point. As more sophisticated tests come into use the upper limit of normal for pressure rise in this hypersensitive group (<15 cm H_2O) may well be revised downwards. Likewise a limit might be set on the bladder capacity permissible for the diagnosis of a hypersensitive disorder to be made. If, for example, the lower limit of the normal range of physiological capacity were agreed at 350 ml for men and 300 ml for women, a level of around 75% of this value might be set—250 ml and 225 ml respectively. Such refinements in definition await scientific agreement though Abrams has also quoted a limit of 250 ml in a study on younger men (Abrams et al. 1981).

is made with the more definite diagnostic techniques available for other diseases. However, the definition of any sensory disorder is made largely by exclusion, a description of negative rather than positive features. As work progresses information will no doubt emerge allowing an even more definitive picture of the disorders to be constructed. Nevertheless, if the diagnostic criteria are correctly and carefully applied, groups of patients emerge who in many respects exhibit remarkable similarities to each other and who may be studied, compared and contrasted in an attempt to understand the underlying pathophysiological and aetiological mechanisms of the sensory disorders.

References

Abrams PH, Farrar DJ, Turner-Warwick RT, Whiteside CG, Feneley RCL (1979) The results of prostatectomy; a symptomatic and urodynamic analysis of 152 patients. J Urol 121:640–642

Abrams PH, Shah PJR, Feneley RCL (1981) Voiding disorders in the young male adult. Urology 18:107–111

Brooks D, Mauder A (1972) Pathogenesis of the urethral syndrome in women and its diagnosis in general practice. Lancet II:893–899

Carson CC, Segura JW, Osborne DM (1980) Evaluation and treatment of the female urethral syndrome. J Urol 124:609–610

Drach GW, Fair WR, Meares EM, Stamey TA (1978) Classification of benign diseases associated with prostatic pain; prostatitis or prostatodynia? J Urol 120:266

George NJR (1978) Influence of lignocaine on bladder instability. Paper presented at the VIIIth meeting of the International Continence Society. Manchester

Higson RH, Smith JC, Hills W (1979) Intravesical lignocaine and detrusor instability. Br J Urol 51: 500–503

Kaplan WE, Firlit CF, Schoenberg HW (1980) The female urethral syndrome: External sphincter spasm as aetiology. J Urol 124:48–49

Kass EH (1955) Chemotherapeutic and antibiotic drugs in the management of infections of the urinary tract. Am J Med 18:764–781

Kass EH, Finland M (1956) Asymptomatic infections of the urinary tract. Trans Assoc Am Physicians 64: 56–64

Keltikangas-Järvinen L, Järvinen H, Lehtonen T (1981) Psychic disturbances in patients with chronic prostatitis. Ann Clin Res 13: 45–49

Lancet (1982) Can kasstigation beat the truth out of the urethral syndrome? Lancet II: 694–695

Mond NC, Percival A, Williams JD, Brumfitt W (1965) Presentation, diagnosis and treatment of urinary tract infections in general practice. Lancet I: 514–516

Nathan PW, Smith MC (1951) The centripetal pathway from the bladder and urethra within the spinal cord. J Neurol Neurosurg Psychiatr 14: 262–280

Rees, DLP, Farhoumand N (1977) Psychiatric aspects of recurrent cystitis in women. Br J Urol 49: 651–658

Segura JW, Opitz JL, Greene LF (1979) Prostatosis, prostatitis or pelvic floor tension myalgia? J Urol 122: 168–169

Stamm WE (1984) Quantitative urine cultures revisited. Eur J Clin Microbiol 3:279–281

Stamm WE, Wagner KF, Ansel R, Alexander ER, Turck M, Counts GW, Holmes KK (1980) Causes of the acute urethral syndrome in women. N Engl J Med 303:409–415

Stamm WE, Counts GW, Running KR, Fihn S, Turck M, Holmes KK (1982) Diagnosis of coliform infection in acutely dysuric women. N Engl J Med 307: 463–468

Chapter 4

Examination and Investigation of Sensory Patients

N.J.R. George and P.H. Powell

A full clinical examination will be required of the patient suspected of having a sensory disorder in order to identify organic pathology, which has first to be excluded as a cause of symptoms (Fig. 4.1). Rectal examination is instructive as an assessment of pelvic floor muscle tension since in many apprehensive patients, particularly males suspected of having prostatodynia, the muscular contraction of the pelvic floor is particularly evident (Segura et al. 1979). Routine haematological and biochemical screening should be undertaken and special attention directed towards the accurate collection of fractionated urine samples. These collections and the necessary urethral swabs for virology and special culture must be carefully planned. The investigation schedule for the collection of specimens from patients referred to the urological out-patient clinic is illustrated in Fig. 4.2. Full descriptions of the investigation techniques are given in the appropriate sections on the urethral syndrome (Chap. 11) and prostatodynia (Chap. 15). Radiographs will be generally unhelpful though chest X-ray and plain abdominal film including kidneys, ureters and bladder should be requested to help exclude other organic disease. Intravenous urography reveals few unexpected abnormalities in these patients but nevertheless it seems likely that the examination will continue to be performed on an empirical basis (Carson et al. 1980).

Cystometric Examination

Cystometric examination is essential for the diagnosis of a sensory disorder (p. 4). The results of such tests are considered in the appropriate sections of the text but brief mention is required of some basic problems involved when undertaking cystometry on these patients.

In any disorder in which discomfort is located to the genital area, the greatest care must be exercised when performing filling and micturating studies which are particularly liable to investigation artefact. Anxiety is probably best allayed during the pre-test interview, at which time the patient can be advised as to the technique and purpose of cystometry. It must be emphasised that this process cannot be rushed and the typical patient commonly requires at least 20 min for

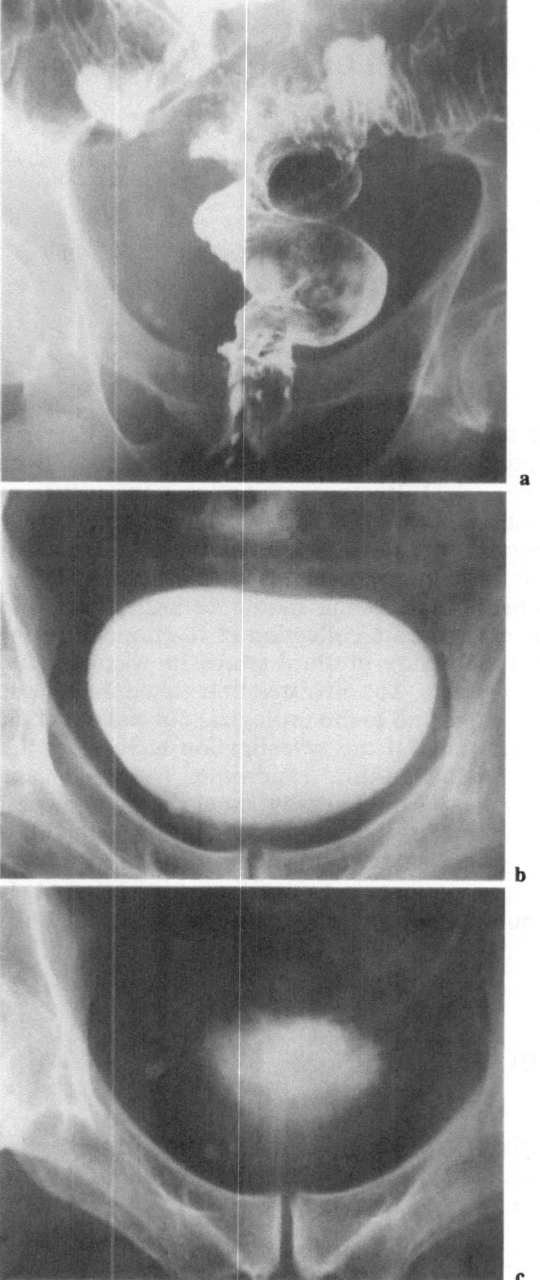

Fig. 4.1a–c. Barium enema and intravenous pyelogram (pre- and post-void films) from man of 54 years with suprapubic ache of 6 months' duration. Loose motions had been present for just 4 weeks prior to presentation. Despite the apparently normal configuration a large diverticular abscess was densely adherent to the posterior and superior aspect of the bladder. The mass was easily felt on bimanual examination.

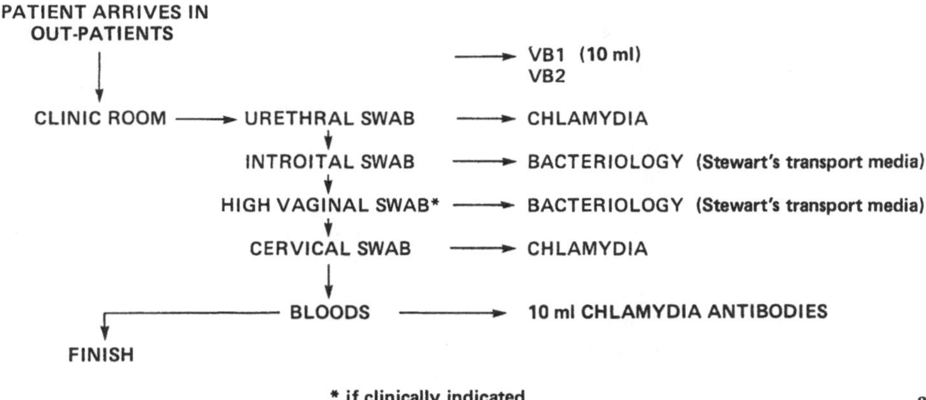

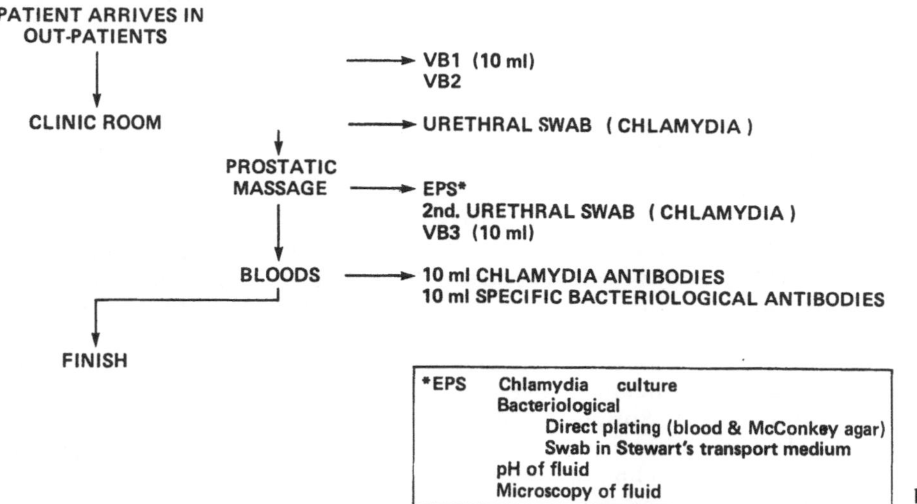

Fig. 4.2. Investigation schedule for **a** male and **b** female patients suspected of harbouring lower urinary tract infection. These schedules require a considerable degree of logistic planning on behalf of the clinic staff.

the history to be satisfactorily obtained in detail. Catheterisation must be expertly performed as pain should be avoided and the patient should be frequently reassured. Few personnel should be present in the examination room and the general atmosphere should be one of warmth and quiet.

Filling studies are particularly difficult in patients with heightened urethral sensation as they are acutely aware of the areas under examination. The investigator must at once inform the patient what is required of him, yet prevent undue anxiety. This balance is difficult to obtain, but with care reliable information will be recorded. Klevmark (1981) considers the usual rates of fluid infusion during cystometry (commonly 60—120 ml/min) to be unphysiologically high. Using a filling rate of 15 ml/min he classified 41 patients with sensory symptoms into two distinct groups according to whether or not their attention could be distracted during bladder filling. Those patients who accepted normal volumes (500 ml) during the test were described as having a 'psychosomatic' sensory problem, in contradistinction to the group with reduced capacity, some of whom had clinical interstitial cystitis.

Voiding studies are best performed in the sitting position with the patient having been given instructions to relax and void normally. Experience demonstrates that many individuals, especially women, find difficulty passing urine in the presence of other people. Hence in conditions in which anxiety and excessive muscle tension are thought to occur, solitary voiding in a quiet room is of importance. For similar reasons, simple pressure and flow studies are to be preferred to the more complex videocystometric examination. To ask an anxious patient to void in front of a camera in the presence of several attendants including doctors, radiographers and nurses is likely to introduce considerable artefact into the test. Iatrogenic 'lack of relaxation' in such patients during videocystometry is likely to outweigh any advantage thought to accrue from visualisation of the lower urinary tract.

Electromyography

Electromyographic evaluation of pelvic floor activity is of potential importance in these patients, many of whom appear to have difficulty in maintaining normal flow (Raz and Smith 1976; Kaplan et al. 1980). It is desirable under these circumstances to know whether the patients are relaxing their sphincter muscles during voiding, but to place invasive electromyographic needle recording electrodes in the perineum of over-aware patients is surely to invite serious experimental artefact. Surface electrodes in part avoid these criticisms, but at the cost of less specific recordings (Kaplan et al. 1980). Thus, both the technical difficulties and practical limitations of electromyography ensure that few sensory patients are investigated by this means. Pelvic floor activity, synergic and dyssynergic voiding is further discussed on p. 160.

Assessment of Anxiety

The assessment of patient anxiety will be difficult in the rushed hospital out-patient interview. Occasionally patients may question whether 'it's all in the mind' or volunteer that they feel their problem may be related to stress at work, but in the majority of cases such self-made observations will not be forthcoming.

Frequency/volume charts (see next paragraph) may be of some help in allowing the patient to recognise his own problem. Specific questions regarding anxiety, depression and other psychological states are best reserved for a specific interview if such a diagnosis is considered likely. Headache, palpitations, somatic anxiety and obsessive phobias will require careful symptom analysis by means of standard psychophysiological methods. Details of such tests are given in Chap. 18.

Frequency/Volume Charts

A chart of micturition frequency and urine volume is essential for the diagnosis and treatment of the sensory disorders (Fig. 4.3a,b). The charts enable the patient to assess urinary tract function prior to meeting the doctor and it is commonly observed that the experience of recording this information allows the patient, often for the first time, to gain some insight into his condition. Patients may comment, for example that they are voiding small amounts throughout the day but hardly at all by night, and such observations may be of therapeutic as well as diagnostic value. It is recognised that the act of self-recording urine volumes for patients whose problem may be psychogenic in origin may well exacerbate their symptoms. Whilst such criticisms are valid, the benefits of frequency/volume charts generally outweigh the disadvantage of additional self-awareness.

Charts often show distinctive patterns which, if correctly interpreted, may be of positive diagnostic significance in the various sensory disorders, especially when the information is used in conjunction with values of bladder capacity obtained under general anaesthetic. The charts reflect the physical and physiological changes that are occurring within the bladder and urethra, and of particular importance in this respect is the compliance of the bladder wall (p. 57). Hence the low compliance of, for example, the post-radiation bladder will demonstrate frequency both by day and night, and the capacity under general anaesthetic will not greatly exceed the conscious volumes (Fig. 4.3c). Patients with interstitial cystitis will show much the same pattern though night volumes may be a little higher (Fig. 6.1b). Some workers give this relentless voiding the rather dramatic title of 'machine-gun' frequency.

Patients with urethral hypersensitivity demonstrate a different voiding pattern and voided volumes may vary widely according to what is occupying the patient's mind (Klevmark 1981). Daytime frequency may be worse at work or it may be more noticeable whilst relaxing depending on what causes the most stress for the patient. At night frequency commonly ceases and the first morning void is of a normal volume (see pp. 96 and 144). Paradoxically these patients may 'hold on' to large volumes of urine if their attention can be distracted or if a concerted conscious effort is made to delay micturition, and the bladder capacity measured under general anaesthetic is almost invariably normal (Powell and Yeates 1982). The generally weak detrusor voiding pressure (see p. 156) in this group can lead to painful retention under some circumstances.

UNIVERSITY OF MANCHESTER

DEPARTMENT OF UROLOGY

Withington Hospital
Nell Lane
West Didsbury
Manchester M20 8LR
Telephone: 445 8111
Extension : 2391

NAME OF PATIENT : ....

HOSPITAL NUMBER : ....

FREQUENCY / VOLUME CHART

Please complete the confidential form overleaf as accurately as possible and:—

a) Bring it with you when you attend the urological out-patients clinic.

b) Send it to Dr .... at the above address.

Please note the time you pass your water, and the volume passed each time. Any measuring jug will do for this purpose.

Obviously there may be times when it is not convenient to measure the volume, for example if you are at work. In that case, record only the time. However, at other times please try to record both.

If you wet yourself at any time, record the time and underneath write the letter "W".

Day time means when you are up. Night time means when you are in bed. An example is given below for you guidance.

EXAMPLE

DAY	TIME / VOLUME (mls) DAY TIME	TIME / VOLUME (mls) NIGHT
1	7am/200 1pm/—* 6pm/400 11pm/300	3am/200 6am/ W**

—* means at work, could not measure volume.

W** means wet at 6 a.m.

Continued overleaf . . . .

a

Fig. 4.3a–c. Frequency volume charts. **a** Front sheet with instructions. **b** Normal 57-year-old male. **c** Woman with radiation bladder disease following treatment for cervical cancer. Note relentless voiding pattern indicative of the 'rigid' bladder wall. Compare with Fig. 6.1b, p. 52. Psychogenic voiding patterns are illustrated in the chapters on the urethral syndrome and on prostatodynia.

IF YOU ARE TO ATTEND FOR AN I.V.P. – THAT IS AN X–RAY OF YOUR KIDNEYS AND BLADDER – DO NOT KEEP ANY RECORD ON THE DATE THAT YOU ATTEND FOR THE X–RAY EXAMINATION.

DAY	TIME / VOLUME DAY TIME (measure volumes in mls, ccs or fl. oz.)	TIME / VOLUME NIGHT TIME
1		
2	6am/650 8/120 2·30/360 5/240 8·30/450 11·30/180	
3	7/900 3pm/240 6·30/360 11·30/540	
4	8·30am/700 1·20pm/240 3/240 6/270 1015/550	
5	6·30am/700 11·45/– 4/– 5·30pm/350 11/350	
6	6·20am/600 10/– 4/– 6·30/540 11pm/180	
7		

ER ♂ age 57. Drinks mod.

Fig. 4.3b

IF YOU ARE TO ATTEND FOR AN I.V.P. – THAT IS AN X–RAY OF YOUR KIDNEYS AND BLADDER – DO NOT KEEP ANY RECORD ON THE DATE THAT YOU ATTEND FOR THE X–RAY EXAMINATION.

DAY	TIME / VOLUME DAY TIME (measure volumes in mls, ccs or fl. oz.)	TIME / VOLUME NIGHT TIME
1	9.00 100 mls 10.45 50 1.30 50 3.00 50 5.00 50 7.00 100 ml 8.00 50 ml	10.00 50 mls 12.00 100 1.30 am 50 3.00 100 5.00 50 6.30 am 50
2	8.30 am 50 mls 11.00 50 12.30 100 2.30 50 4.00 50 6.00 50 8.00 50	10.00 pm 50 12.00 100 2.30 50 4.00 100 5.00 100 6.30 200
3	10 am 50 mls 1.00 20 2.30 50 5.00 100 8.00 50 mls	10.00 50 mls 1.00 am 100 2.00 100 5.00 200 7.00 100 mls 8am 100
4	9am 50 mls 11.00 100 1.00 100 2.00 100 4pm 100 6.00 100 8.00 50	10.00 100 mls 12.00 100 mls 1.30am 100 mls 3am 100 mls 5.30 100 7.30 100
5	9.00am - 50 mls 10.00 50 12.00 100 3.00 100 4.00 100 7.00 100	9.00pm 100 mls 10.00 50 12.00 100 2 am 100 5.00 100 7.00 100 8.00 100
6	10 am 50 mls 12.00 100 2.00 100 4pm 100 6.00 50 7.00 100	9.pm 100 11.00 100 1.00 100 3.00 100 6.am 100 mls
7	8am 100 mls 9.30 50 11.30 100 1.pm 100 2.30 100 4.00 50 6.00 100 7.00 50	9.pm -100 mls 11.00 100 2.00 100 5.00 100 7am 100 mls

♀ age 68. Bed @ 10pm.

Fig. 4.3c

Assessment of Bladder and Urethral Sensation

The sensory perception of the bladder depends on exteroceptive and proprioceptive (pressure–volume) receptors (Hald 1969). These receptors are not adequately assessed by standard urodynamic investigation techniques which usually measure detrusor stretch responses, muscle strength and motor activity (Kiesswetter 1977). Before the introduction of the mucosal electrosensitivity test, the assessment of sensory bladder function was limited to recordings of post-void residual urine, first desire to micturate (FDM) and total bladder capacity, together with an analysis of the form of the inflow cystometrogram.

Frimodt-Moller (1972) first described the technique of mucosal electrosensitivity as a method of evaluating bladder sensation. In this method a thin silver wire was passed into the bladder which had previously been filled with 200 ml of saline. A stimulator delivered constant current square wave impulses of 1 ms duration and frequency 2.5 Hz to the wire, and by changing the amplitude of the current the patient registered a sensation of 'burning' or 'tickling'. The lowest amplitude of current able to produce this sensation was recorded as the electrical perception threshold of the bladder. Kiesswetter (1977) modified this technique and constructed a sensitivity catheter on which were mounted both positive and negative stimulating electrodes. Thus it was possible not only to reduce the quantity of the stimulating current, but also to assess bladder and urethral sensation independently by re-positioning the catheter within the urethra. Several types of sensitivity catheter design have subsequently been investigated by Powell and Feneley (1980). Refinements in the positioning of the electrodes in relation to either the drainage holes or balloon of the catheter enables accurate placement in the urethra (Fig. 4.4).

The measurement of electrosensitivity is usually performed after the completion of a standard water-fill cystogram, allowing the patients to become accustomed to the presence of the urethral catheter. Although the stimulation parameters have varied with different investigators, the technique of recording the sensitivity threshold has been basically similar in all the reported series (Murray 1982), and has been shown to give reproducible results (Opsomer et al. 1983).

Sensory Innervation of the Posterior Urethra

It is not yet clear whether bladder and urethral sensation are mediated by proprioceptive or exteroceptive receptors and pathways. Keele (1966) suggests that receptors for recording pain register sensations of 'burning' or 'tingling' at a lower stimulus than that required to produce pain, and therefore it is probable that bladder and urethral electrosensitivity are exteroceptive measurements. However, it will be apparent from the description of the receptors and afferent nerve pathways given on p. 14 that there must be an area in the region of the posterior urethra that constitutes a watershed between exteroceptive afferents carried in the pelvic nerve and those carried in the pudendal nerve.

This divide, and the lack of information concerning its location, constitutes a basic problem for both clinician and urodynamic investigator. Tests of urethral

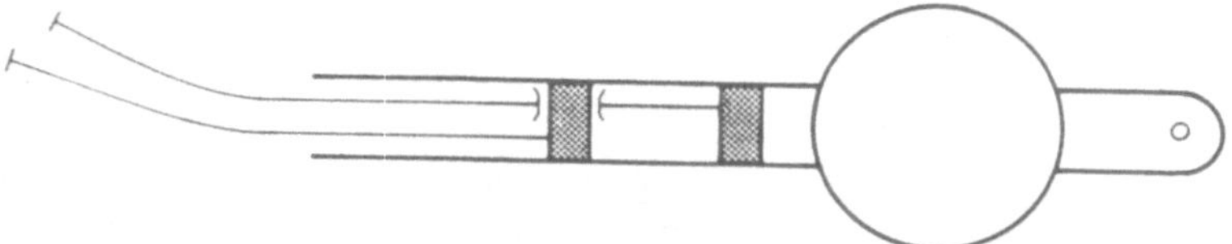

Fig. 4.4. Catheter for measuring urethral sensitivity. *Stippled areas*, platinum stimulating electrodes.

sensitivity (Kiesswetter 1977; Powell and Feneley 1980) in which a catheter with stimulating electrodes is placed in the posterior urethra may effect a response by either route. If such stimulation is in fact passing via the pudendal nerve the test will not involve an *essential* pathway of the micturition reflex, and in this respect it is notable that abnormalities of urethral sensation may be partially abolished by pudendal nerve blockade (Raz and Smith 1976). However, recent studies, in which results from such tests have been equated with the first desire to micturate assessed by urodynamic methods, suggest that at least some electrosensitivity afferent activity might be passing by the pelvic nerve, reflecting an important component of the storage/voiding cycle of the bladder (Murray 1982). Thus the results of electrosensitivity testing of the posterior urethra require interpretation not only in the light of technical factors such as current stimulus intensity but also as regards the possible routes of afferent traffic and the basically subjective nature of the response in the patient groups under study.

Alterations in bladder and urethral electrosensitivity have been described in various forms of lower urinary tract dysfunction including neurological disease and detrusor instability (Powell and Feneley 1980). In addition, a positive correlation has been demonstrated between urethral (Powell and Feneley 1980) and bladder (Opsomer et al. 1983) sensation, when compared with the cystometric measurements of FDM and bladder capacity. It would thus appear that the measurement of bladder and urethral electrosensitivity may provide a reproducible and semi-objective assessment of sensory abnormality in lower urinary tract dysfunction.

Microbiological Considerations

The relevant bacteriology and virology concerned with the urethral syndrome (Chap. 10) and prostatitis (Chap. 15) are discussed elsewhere. Certain basic points, however, require emphasis if the clinician is to be successful in his efforts to diagnose and distinguish the sensory disorders from other dysfunctions of the lower urinary tract.

Attention to detail is likely to be of importance in making these diagnoses and the interested clinician will undoubtedly familiarise himself with the basic bacteriological skills of plating, microscopy and other techniques. The logistic problems concerned with specimen collection have been previously mentioned

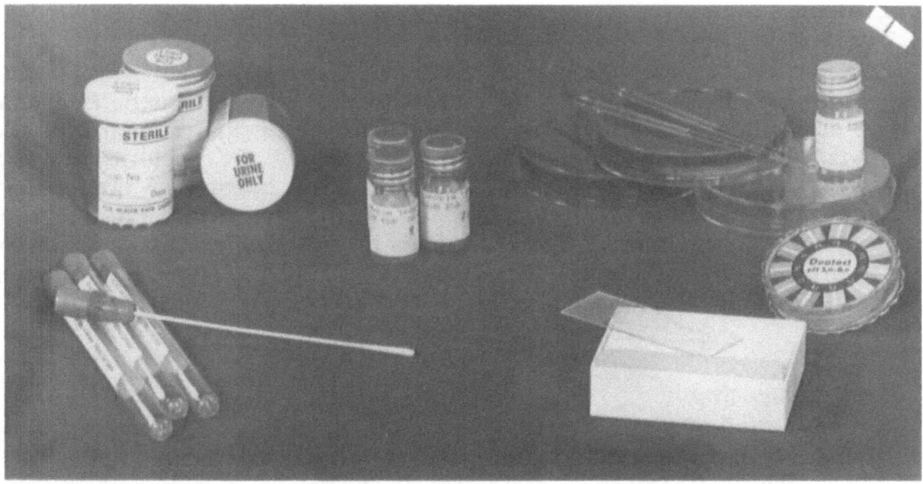

Fig. 4.5. Trolley prepared for prostatodynia clinic. Specific swabs and medium for chlamydia culture, fractional urine pots, pH papers and culture plates for direct plating of specimens.

(see p. 31). There will be certain minimum requirements as regards equipment which must be readily available when studies are to be performed either in the clinic or operating theatre. Figure 4.5 illustrates a typical trolley prepared for an out-patient clinic dealing with cases of prostatodynia. Attempting to make a diagnosis without this facility ready and available is to admit defeat almost before the start of the investigation. A nurse helper who is familiar with the collection techniques and who can check culture media, swabs, plates and other equipment is an invaluable member of the clinic team. Specimens should be transported direct to the appropriate laboratories and overnight storage avoided. For this reason, and the fact that the schedules are somewhat tiring for both doctor and nurse, investigations are best performed during the early part of the clinic or operating list.

Biopsy Requirements

Similar planning must be applied to the collection of biopsy specimens for morphological analysis and it is essential that advance notice is given to the personnel involved so as to prepare materials and fixative appropriate to the case.

Examination Under Anaesthetic

It is helpful to examine the sensory patient under both local and general anaesthetic.

Local Anaesthetic

Studies with local anaesthetic blocking agents may be of assistance in the diagnosis and management of some patients with sensory disorders. Pudendal nerve anaesthesia with either short or long acting agents may demonstrate the importance of selective neurological components of the micturition reflex (Emmett et al. 1948; Raz and Smith 1976). Temporary benefit may occasionally be obtained in patients with urethral hypersensitivity after such blockage. Local anaesthetic placed upon the trigone or within the posterior urethra may modify detrusor behaviour (George 1978; Higson et al. 1979), abolishing catheter sensation and increasing residual urine after micturition.

General Anaesthetic

Examination under general anaesthesia is often the last, but not the least important diagnostic test to be performed on the patient suspected of having a sensory disorder. The surgeon will always seek first to exclude organic disease by all appropriate means. Following routine collection of microbiological samples the urethra and all regions of the bladder will be thoroughly inspected.

It is important that some standardisation be introduced regarding the physical conditions under which the bladder is inspected and biopsied. For some years Powell and Yeates (1982) have routinely observed the lower urinary tract utilising a 10 cm head of pressure within the irrigating apparatus; in this way it was considered that 'physiological' rather than 'distension' conditions applied to the examination. Under these circumstances it was possible to identify two distinct groups of 'sensory' patients, those with a normal and those with reduced capacity under anaesthetic (see also p. 100). Workers in the field of interstitial cystitis have, however, agreed on 80 cm as the optimal height of the irrigating fluid above the suprapubic level (see p. 59). It is evident that standardisation along agreed lines is essential if results from different series of patients are to be compared and contrasted with one another.

Depth of anaesthesia is a further variable which remains very difficult to quantify in any given clinical situation. Use of different inhalation or injectable agents on patients within single series must be expected to lead to significant variation in tolerated bladder capacity. There seems at present no simple method of overcoming these difficulties.

References

Carson CC, Segura JW, Osborne DM (1980) Evaluation and treatment of the female urethral syndrome. J Urol 124:609–610

Emmett JL, Daut RV, Dunn JH (1948) Role of the external urethral sphincter in the normal bladder and cord bladder. J Urol 59:439–454

Frimodt-Møller C (1972) A new method for quantitative evaluation of bladder sensibility. Scand J Urol Nephrol 6 (Suppl. 15):135–142

George NJR (1978) Influence of lignocaine on bladder instability. Paper presented at the VIIIth meeting of the International Continence Society. Manchester

Hald T (1969) Neurogenic dysfunction of the urinary bladder. Thesis, University of Copenhagen

Higson RH, Smith JC, Hills W (1979) Intravesical lignocaine and detrusor instability. Br J Urol 51:500–503

Kaplan WE, Firlit CF, Schoenberg HW (1980) The female urethral syndrome: external sphincter spasm as etiology. J Urol 124:48–49

Keele CA (1966) Touch, heat and pain. Ciba Foundation Symposium, Churchill, London

Kiesswetter H (1977) Mucosal sensory threshold of the urinary bladder and urethra measured electrically. Urol Int 32:437–448

Klevmark B (1981) Hyperactive neurogenic bladder studied with physiological filling rates. Scand J Urol Nephrol (Suppl) 60: 55–56

Murray K (1982) Urethral sensitivity—An integral component of the storage phase of the micturation cycle. Neurol Urodyn 1:193–197

Opsomer RJ, Gerstenberg TC, Klarskov P, Hald T (1983) The electric sensibility threshold in the bladder and the urethra. Paper presented at the XIIIth meeting of the International Continence Society

Powell PH, Feneley RCL (1980) The role of urethral sensation in clinical urology. Br J Urol 52: 539–541

Powell PH, Yeates WK (1982) The clinical value of bladder capacity measurement at physiological pressure under anaesthesia Br J Urol 54:650–652

Raz S, Smith RB (1976) External sphincter spasticity syndrome in female patients. J Urol 115:443–446

Segura JW, Opitz JL, Greene LF (1979) Prostatosis, prostatitis or pelvic floor tension myalgia? J Urol 122:168–169

Section 2

Interstitial Cystitis

Chapter 5

Historical Perspective

R.J. Barnard

Hunner (1915) first described a rare type of bladder ulcer in a group of eight female patients whose average age was 37 years and whose symptoms included frequency, nocturia, urgency and suprapubic pain for periods up to 17 years. Urine examination was unhelpful but cystoscopy revealed that all had ulcers or smooth white scars with surrounding hyperaemia in the vault of the bladder. Examination of surgically removed specimens demonstrated rather non-specific changes of absent epithelium, chronic granulation tissue and capillaries packed with leucocytes. This condition was given the name 'submucous ulcer' of the bladder by Bumpus in 1921.

Previous reports along similar lines had been made at the beginning of the century by Nitze (1907), who described a 'cystitis parenchymatosa', and earlier still in 1836 Mercier had documented spontaneous bladder rupture associated with ulcers. However, in most of these cases lower urinary tract obstruction and infection appear to have been the relevant underlying abnormalities. The term 'interstitial cystitis' was coined by A. J. C. Skene, whose monograph on female bladder and urethral disease was published in 1878.

The primary symptoms of this condition are frequency of urination, persistent urgency and suprapubic pain—complaints common to many urological disorders. It is not surprising, therefore, that over the years many reports linking these symptoms to a range of cystoscopic appearances have been made. The classical findings of a contracted, scarred bladder which splits and bleeds on distension are, in the absence of other histologically defined conditions such as tuberculosis or carcinoma, reasonably easy to recognise. By contrast hyperaemia, petechiae and free bleeding in a bladder of normal capacity are less specific signs which may be related either to vesical disease or to extraneous factors such as the pressure of the irrigation fluid used during cystoscopy. Hand (1949) reported that of 223 patients diagnosed as having interstitial cystitis on clinical grounds, only 29 had the classical cystoscopic appearances associated with the condition. It seems unlikely that mechanical or hydraulic factors alone could explain this apparent discrepancy between symptoms and signs, and the advent of urodynamics, combined with routine bladder biopsy, might be expected to throw some light on the aetiology of the disorder found in patients with atypical symptom complexes.

The absence of clear-cut pathognomonic markers by which to diagnose interstitial cystitis has lead in the past to a variety of theories concerning the aetiology of the disease. Bumpus (1921) considered the signs to be indicative of streptococcal infection but by careful study Hanash and Pool (1979) excluded bacterial, viral and fungal infection as causes of the symptom complex. Herbst (1937) considered that the typical lesions could be due to trauma whilst Powell (1945) implicated lymphatic obstruction in the pathogenesis of the disease.

Early questions concerning the role of autoimmune mechanisms were raised when Fister (1938) noted a similarity between the pathological changes found in both interstitial cystitis and systemic lupus erythematosus. Since that date Bohne et al. (1962) and other workers (see below) have variously described abnormal serological findings, none of which, however, have been found to be specific for interstitial cystitis.

It has been suggested that the mast cell may serve as a marker for interstitial cystitis. Simmons (1961) described the presence of these cells in the bladder wall of patients with clinical evidence of the disorder and suggested treatment with antihistamines. Although Messing and Stamey (1978) disputed the validity and specificity of this observation, the mast cell has continued to excite the interest of workers in the field of the 'suprapubic discomfort syndrome' (Larsen et al. 1982).

At the present time research into this enigmatic condition continues to be hampered by a lack of exact diagnostic criteria and the possibility that the disorder may result from a number of different aetiological factors. In the following chapters, whilst due consideration is given to the broad spectrum of suprapubic disorders, attention is focussed on interstitial cystitis as it presents in its most typical form.

References

Bohne AW, Hodson JM, Rebuck JW, Reinhard RE (1962) An abnormal leukocyte response in interstitial cystitis. J Urol 88:387–391

Bumpus HG (1921) Submucous ulcer of the bladder in the male. J Urol 5:249–253

Fister GM (1938) Similarity of interstitial cystitis to lupus erythematosus. J Urol 40: 37–51

Hanash KA, Pool TL (1969) Interstitial cystitis in men. J Urol 102: 427–428

Hand JR (1949) Interstitial cystitis: Report of 223 cases (204 women and 19 men). J Urol 61: 291–310

Herbst RH, Baumrucher GO, German KL (1937) Elusive ulcer (Hunner) of the bladder with an experimental study of the etiology. Am J Surg 38:152–167

Hunner GL (1915) A rare type of bladder ulcer in women: report of cases. Boston Med Surg J 172:660–664

Larsen S, Thompson SA, Hald T, Barnard RJ, Gilpin CJ, Dixon JS, Gosling JA (1982) Mast cells in interstitial cystitis. Br J Urol 54: 283–286

Mercier LA (1836) Memoire sur certaines perforations spontenées de la vessie non dèscrites jusqu'a ce jour. Gaz Med Paris 4:257

Messing EM, Stamey TA (1978) Interstitial cystitis: Early diagnosis, pathology and treatment. Urology 12:381–392

Nitze M (1907) Lehrbuch de Kystoskopie: Ihre Technik und Klinische Bedeutung. JE Bergman, Berlin, p 410

Powell TO (1945) Studies on the etiology of Hunner ulcer. J Urol 53:823–835

Simmons JL (1961) Interstitial cystitis: An explanation for the beneficial effect of an antihistamine. J Urol 85:149–155

Skene AJC (1878) Diseases of bladder and urethra in men. Wm. Wood, New York, p 167

Chapter 6

Clinical Symptom Complex

T. Hald and M. Holm-Bentzen

Introduction

An essential prerequisite to the diagnosis of a particular disease is that the condition conforms to clearly defined criteria. Interstitial cystitis is an example of a condition where few specific criteria have been established and the diagnosis often relies upon the experience and personal bias of the physician. Thus a collection of symptoms and signs which would be acceptable as a basis for the diagnosis in one clinic may not be considered appropriate in another. This variability has hampered progress, particularly since the scarcity of these patients emphasises the need to pool data from different centres in order to identify common features and to evaluate differing forms of treatment.

Incidence and Natural History

There is no agreement as to the specific histological, serological or clinical features of this symptom complex and consequently essential criteria to which one can refer for comparative purposes do not exist. At present, therefore, the diagnosis is based upon the patient's symptoms, a complete examination including cystoscopy having first been performed in order to exclude all other forms of recognised bladder disease (BMJ 1972; Walsh 1978; Messing and Stamey 1978) (Table 6.1).

The incidence of interstitial cystitis is difficult to assess although Oravisto (1975) estimated its occurrence in Helsinki at 18.1 per 100 000 women whilst a survey in London found only 27 cases amongst over 17 000 urological registrations drawn from a large urban population (Kinder and Smith 1958). Changes thought to be typical of interstitial cystitis have been observed in the bladder of patients with autoimmune diseases (see Table 6.2) and such reports have lead to speculation as to the role of immunological factors in the disorder (Silk 1970; Oravisto et al. 1970). Allergic reactions were noted to occur in as many as 26% of patients with interstitial cystitis (Oravisto 1980).

Table 6.1. Differential diagnosis in interstitial cystitis

Abacterial cystitis (mycoplasma, virus, trichomonas, yeast)
Chronic bacterial cystitis
Irradiation cystitis
Cyclophosphamide cystitis
Eosinophilic cystitis
Allergic cystitis
Tuberculous cystitis
Bilharzia cystitis
Syphilitic affection
Carcinoma in situ
Bladder cancer
Malacoplakia
Leucoplakia
Leukaemic infiltrations
Granulomatous cystitis

Table 6.2. Autoimmune diseases reported to have been associated with interstitial cystitis

Polyarteritis nodosa
Systemic lupus erythematosus
Rheumatoid arthritis
Scleroderma
Ulcerative colitis
Boeck's sarcoidosis
Hashimoto's thyroiditis

The natural history of interstitial cystitis is variable and difficult to project (Hand 1949). The onset is commonly subacute rather than insidious and full development of the classical symptom complex takes place over a relatively short time (Oravisto 1975; Messing and Stamey 1978). Fewer than 10% of cases progress rapidly towards a small shrunken bladder whilst the majority continue with a relatively normal or slightly subnormal bladder capacity. The absence of specific pathognomonic markers also precludes determination of spontaneous remission rates of the disease, and figures of 10%–15% quoted in the literature should be interpreted with caution (Oravisto 1975).

Clinical History

The most important symptoms of the patient with 'classical' interstitial cystitis are pain, frequency, nocturia and urgency for fear of suprapubic discomfort (sensory urgency). It has already been noted that these symptoms are common to many urological disorders and thus particular care is required when eliciting this history, which may be considered to be characteristic rather than pathognomonic of the disease. *Pain* is usually experienced in the suprapubic region, but occasionally radiates into the loins, particularly when the bladder is full. In most cases voiding relieves the pain, but in the latter phases of severe disease the pain may become dissociated from the micturition cycle and be present continuously. Urethral discomfort and dysuria are occasionally described but these symptoms are rather non-specific and usually not of diagnostic importance. *Nocturia* is a particularly common symptom, the patient being awakened by a strong and often painful desire to void. This relentless frequency results from a reduction in bladder capacity and usually, despite attempting to restrict fluids in the evening, the patient cannot avoid the constant need to pass urine during the night. By contrast, in patients in whom a psychoneurotic aetiology is suspected, nocturia is rarely a dominating symptom (see pp. 92–142). *Diurnal frequency* and urgency (due to suprapubic pain) is common in interstitial cystitis but these non-specific symptoms are difficult to evaluate.

Reference to a self-recorded voiding chart completed during a period of 3 or 4 days is often very helpful in quantifying these symptoms (Fig. 6.1) As might be expected, those patients most afflicted with daytime frequency suffer from severe nocturia. Incontinence is not a common complaint in patients with interstitial cystitis.

Other Symptoms

Of patients with interstitial cystitis 20%–30% experience episodes of macroscopic haematuria (Messing and Stamey 1978). The presence of 'smokey' urine or overt blood in the urine at the termination of the stream, particularly after delaying micturition, is a sign of diagnostic significance. At cystoscopy such terminal bleeding may be seen to be the result of haemorrhage from linear cracks in the bladder mucosa (see below). It might be expected that as urinary

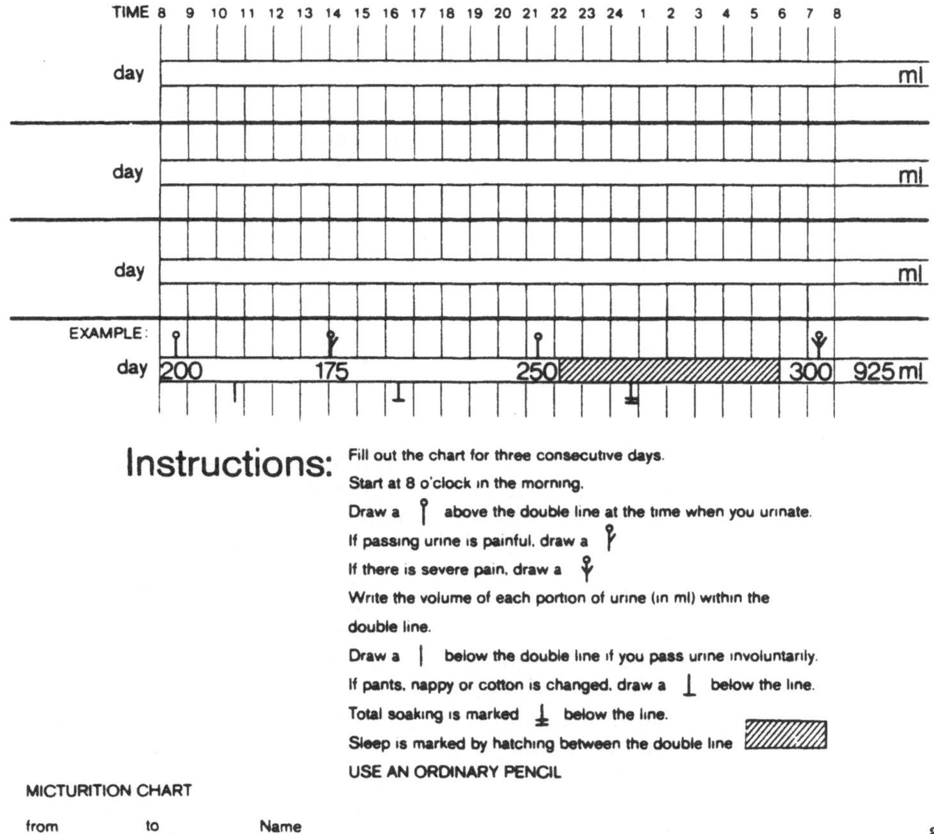

Fig. 6.1a,b. A voiding chart is helpful in substantiating the patient's history. **a** Chart used in Copenhagen. **b** (*next page*) Completed chart from Manchester, female aged 55. Note 'relentless' voiding pattern both by day and night.

IF YOU ARE TO ATTEND FOR AN I.V.P. – THAT IS AN X–RAY OF YOUR KIDNEYS AND BLADDER – DO NOT KEEP ANY RECORD ON THE DATE THAT YOU ATTEND FOR THE X–RAY EXAMINATION.

DAY	TIME / VOLUME DAY TIME (measure volumes in mls, ccs or fl. oz.)	TIME / VOLUME NIGHT TIME
1		
2	9am 100 ml 10.45 100 1.30 75 4pm 75 5.30/50 7.00 100 8.30 75	10.30 50 12 midnight 100 1.00 am 75 2.30 75 4.30 50 6.00 75
3	8am 50 10.30 100 12.00 100 2.30pm 75 4 75 5.30 50 7.30 75	10pm 50 11.30 100 2.00 75 3.30 75 5.00 100 6.00 150
4	8.30 am 75 12.00 100 2.30 50 4.30 100 7pm 75 9.00 50	10pm 100 12.30 75 2.30 100 5am 75 7.00 100

Fig. 6.1b

tract infection occurs frequently in adult women (Stamey 1974), significant bacteruria would be common amongst patients with interstitial cystitis, of whom 90% are female (Oravisto 1975). Therefore, although the finding of urinary tract infection in the patient's history does not exclude the possibility of interstitial cystitis, the diagnosis cannot be reached unless the patient presents with typical symptoms at a time when the urine is found to be sterile (Badenoch 1971; Collan et al. 1976; Herbst et al. 1937). Psychological problems are rare even in the well established cases of interstitial cystitis although distress may be caused by the very frequent need to void. Physical examination is often negative although suprapubic and vaginal tenderness may sometimes be noted (Badenoch 1971).

In summary, the patient in whom the diagnosis of interstitial cystitis is likely will usually be a female, between 30 and 70 years of age, with a rapid development of suprapubic pain on bladder filling, nocturia, frequency, sensory urgency without severe dysuria and occasional episodes of macroscopic haematuria which will occur particularly at the end of the stream. The diagnosis is less likely in males (Hanash and Pool 1969) and children (Geist and Antolak 1970) although it is important to recognise that interstitial cystitis may occasionally occur in these populations.

Techniques of Investigation

Biochemical Investigation

Neither blood tests nor serological investigation can lead with certainty to the diagnosis. There have been many reports concerning allergic and immunological manifestations in patients suspected of having interstitial cystitis. Oravisto et al. (1970) reported elevated antinuclear antibody titres in 85% of cases, but this finding has not been confirmed in unequivocal cases studied by Hald and co-workers (1982, unpublished observations) or Messing and Stamey (1978). Bohne et al. (1962) reported an abnormal leucocyte response in skin windows of patients with interstitial cystitis, whilst Silk (1970) found bladder antibodies in the serum of 9 out of 18 patients. In this context Gordon et al. (1973) found a specific response to antigens present within the patient's own bladder.

Lose et al. (1983) found an elevated serum and urine eosinophilic cationic protein concentration in patients with interstitial cystitis and noted a decrease in levels following heparin treatment. Eosinophilic cationic protein is not excreted via the kidneys and its presence in urine in interstitial cystitis seems likely to be due to secretion from the bladder wall. In selected cases further specialised tests aimed at collagen disease may be appropriate.

The use of several serological tests has failed to assist the diagnosis of interstitial cystitis (Table 6.3). However, a lymphocyte migration test (Fig. 6.2) and lymphocytotoxicity study using bladder mucosal cells as the antigen (Fig. 6.3) has enabled a distinction to be made between a group of interstitial cystitis patients and controls. At present it is questionable as to whether these tests will

Table 6.3. Serotests performed in the diagnosis of 13 cases of interstitial cystitis

Test	Number of patients with abnormal/ elevated findings
Orosomucoid	
Haptoglobin	
Transferrin	1
Fibrinogen	1
IgG	1
IgA	
IgM	
IgE	
C-reactive protein	1
Rose-Waaler	
Organ-unspecific ANF	
Organ-specific ANF	1
DNA	
Complement C_{1q}	1
Complement C_3	1
Complement C_4	3
Complement C_5	

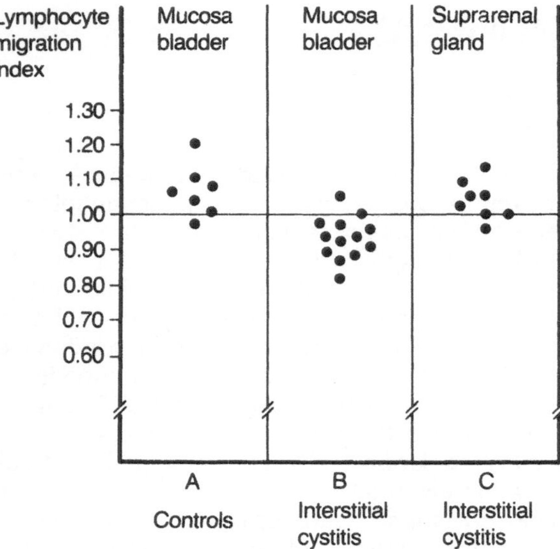

Fig. 6.2. *A*, Lymphocytes from normal controls tested against bladder mucosa extracts. *B*, Lymphocytes from patient with interstitial cystitis tested against bladder mucosa extracts. *C*, Lymphocytes from patient with interstitial cystitis tested against adrenal tissue extracts.
Values <1.00 indicate inhibited lymphocyte migration. The results show a statistically significant ($P<0.01$) reduced lymphocyte migration for interstitial cystitis patients when tested against bladder mucosa in a concentration of 25 μg/ml. (Hald et al. 1982, unpublished observations)

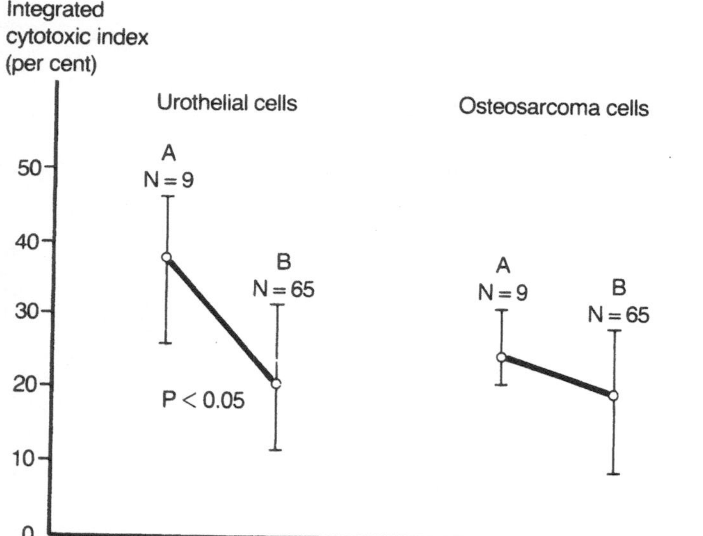

Fig. 6.3. Lymphocytes from nine patients with interstitial cystitis (*A*) and 65 controls (*B*) tested in a tissue culture of urothelial cells and a line of osteosarcoma cells. The lymphocytes of interstitial cystitis patients exhibited a toxic influence on the urothelial cell lines but not on the osteosarcoma cells ($P<0.05$). (By courtesy of Dr. M. Vilien)

provide diagnostic information in individual cases. However, they have provided positive evidence that a cellular rather than a humoral response is involved in the disorder process.

Analysis of Urine

Urinary tract infection must be identified, and repeated cultures may be necessary to isolate all pathogens, including yeasts. Urethral and vaginal cultures for *Chlamydia trachomatis* and *Trichomonas vaginalis* should be performed. In areas where tuberculosis, syphilis and bilharzia are frequently encountered the appropriate investigations are warranted. Urine microscopy may reveal the presence of both red and white cells in the urine but the characteristic finding is the presence of thread-like structures as illustrated in Fig. 6.4. The composition of these threads is at present unknown.

Finally it is important to exclude carcinoma in situ by means of urine cytology (Utz and Zinke 1974).

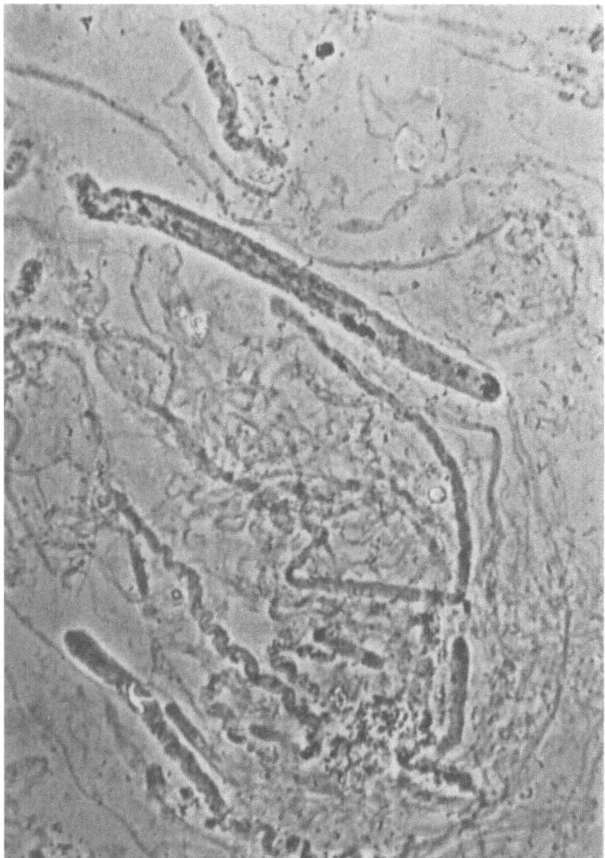

Fig. 6.4. 'Slimy threads' revealed on urinalysis of patient with interstitial cystitis.

Urodynamic Investigation

Urodynamic studies are not considered essential in order to establish the diagnosis. However, some groups of patients may have cystometry performed as part of the general investigation before the presence of interstitial cystitis is confirmed. The investigation is often very uncomfortable for these patients as a result of suprapubic bladder pain during filling and severe sensory urgency may be demonstrated, with the first desire to micturate being experienced at low bladder volumes (Dunn et al. 1977). Average bladder capacity is reduced although some patients may occasionally have normal cystometric capacities. The majority of patients with interstitial cystitis have bladders which do not exhibit phasic unstable waves, though the finding of this abnormality does not exclude the diagnosis.

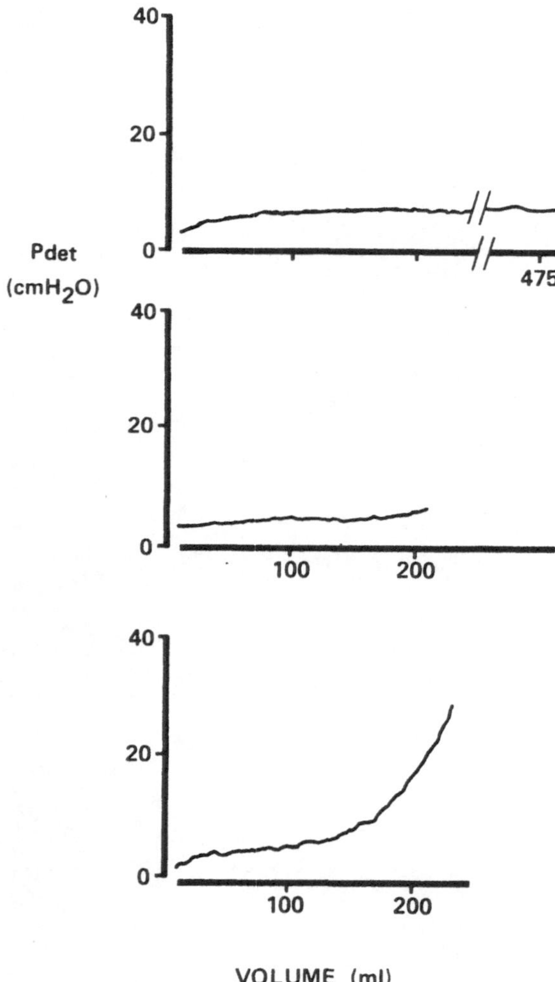

Fig. 6.5a

Bladder Compliance and Interstitial Cystitis

The compliance of the bladder expresses the relationship between increments of pressure and volume within the viscus. The physical changes that are observed are largely due to the properties of the bladder wall itself. Low compliance implies an altered volume/pressure ratio such that an abnormal pressure rise occurs within the bladder for a given increment in volume; the bladder wall may be considered to be more 'stiff' or 'unyielding' than normal.

Patients with interstitial cystitis usually have inflow cystometrograms demonstrating normal compliance. However, the degree to which the patient is prepared to suffer pain is important, and a stoical person may experience quite severe discomfort before insisting that the test be halted (Fig. 6.5a). Under these circumstances the compliance will be seen to be lessened (Fig. 6.5b) and indeed under anaesthetic these patients will, of course, all demonstrate low compliant bladders—this being the essential raison d'être of cystodistension therapy for interstitial cystitis.

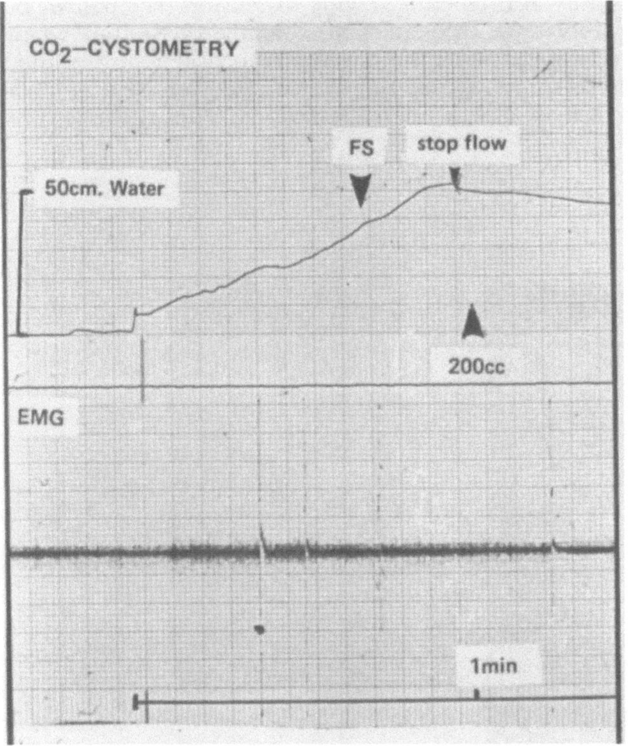

Fig. 6.5a,b. Bladder compliance in patients with interstitial cystitis. **a** Normal compliance is seen both in normal controls (*above*) and in the majority of patients with interstitial cystitis (*middle*). Reduced compliance (*below*) may be demonstrated during standard water cystometrography if the patient can withstand the pain arising from the shrunken bladder (fill rate 60 ml/min). **b** Decreased compliance observed during an inflow cystometrogram with carbon dioxide (fill rate 200 cc/min).

Radiological Investigations

Intravenous urography is indicated in those cases of interstitial cystitis in which the bladder is contracted. In many such patients normal findings will be recorded although a proportion of patients may have signs of obstructive uropathy secondary to constriction of the intramural ureter. Vesico-ureteric reflux may occasionally be observed though voiding cysto-urethrograms are not indicated as a routine investigation procedure.

Cystoscopy

Cystoscopic examination is of particular importance in making the diagnosis of interstitial cystitis (Hand 1949; Kinder and Smith 1958; Oravisto et al. 1970; Messing and Stamey 1978). The most consistent finding is bleeding *on refilling* of the bladder following the initial inspection. Bleeding may take the form of petechial haemorrhage, ecchymoses or free bleeding from vessels, and may be seen in up to 90% of patients with interstitial cystitis. However, patients with a non-specific chronic cystitis may also bleed following distension (see below, p. 22). Classical ulcers are rarely seen (Messing and Stamey 1978), but when present are linear and white in appearance and resemble mucosal fissures rather than true ulcers (Fig. 6.6). In some regions the mucosa is often of a reddish appearance whilst in others it may appear relatively normal. These changes are

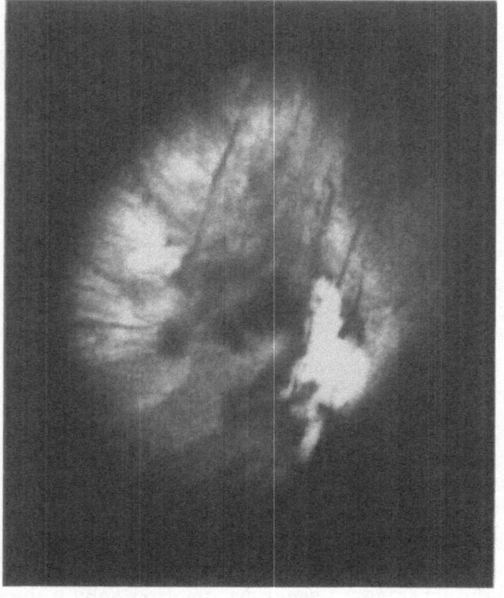

Fig. 6.6. Hunner's ulcer. The linear white fissure is observed on refilling of the bladder; blood is seen streaming away from adjacent ecchymoses.

pronounced in the dome or lateral of the bladder and are rarely seen on the trigone. Debris may be attached to the urothelial surface or observed floating within the bladder lumen.

Cystoscopic Procedure

Valuable information at cystoscopy may be obtained by observing the following procedure.

The bladder is filled with irrigation solution at a pressure of 80 cm of water. After 1 min the bladder is drained and the volume measured to record the capacity under these controlled conditions. This volume provides a measure of the degree of bladder wall fibrosis. Following the initial drainage the bladder is refilled and examined for the presence and sites of petechiae (Fig. 6.7b), ecchymoses (Fig. 6.7c) or free bleeding. Mucosal cracks and fissures, if present, are best observed at the second bladder filling. Further distension is recommended by some authors, but it may be that the features observed on the initial refilling become less specific after each subsequent distension. At the conclusion of cystoscopy deep biopsies are obtained to include detrusor muscle (Fig. 6.8).

Biopsy Procedure

The risks in obtaining deep bladder biopsy can be minimised by adhering to a standard technique. Bladder perforation is unlikely if samples are obtained from the lateral walls with the bladder almost empty. Under these conditions the bladder wall is thick and a standard cold cup biopsy is unlikely to extend through the thickness of the bladder wall. When adequate detrusor muscle specimens are obtained the reticular structure of the detrusor muscle is evident in the depths of the biopsy site (Fig. 6.9). Bleeding vessels are coagulated and the irrigation fluid should be clear at the termination of the procedure. Post-operatively catheterisation is usually maintained for 24 hours.

The number of biopsies depends upon the diversity of the histological methods being employed. Two biopsies will be sufficient but if electron microscopy or immunofluorescent microscopy and biochemical assay are to be performed, six or eight biopsies may be required and these can be taken from random areas of the dome and lateral walls of the bladder.

Concluding Remarks—Value of Diagnostic Methods

In Fig. 6.10 the methods which are of value in reaching the diagnosis of interstitial cystitis have been summarised. The diagnosis should rely on the patient's history, cystoscopic evaluation and the histological features of the bladder biopsies. Other investigations may aid, but are not able to confirm the precise diagnosis.

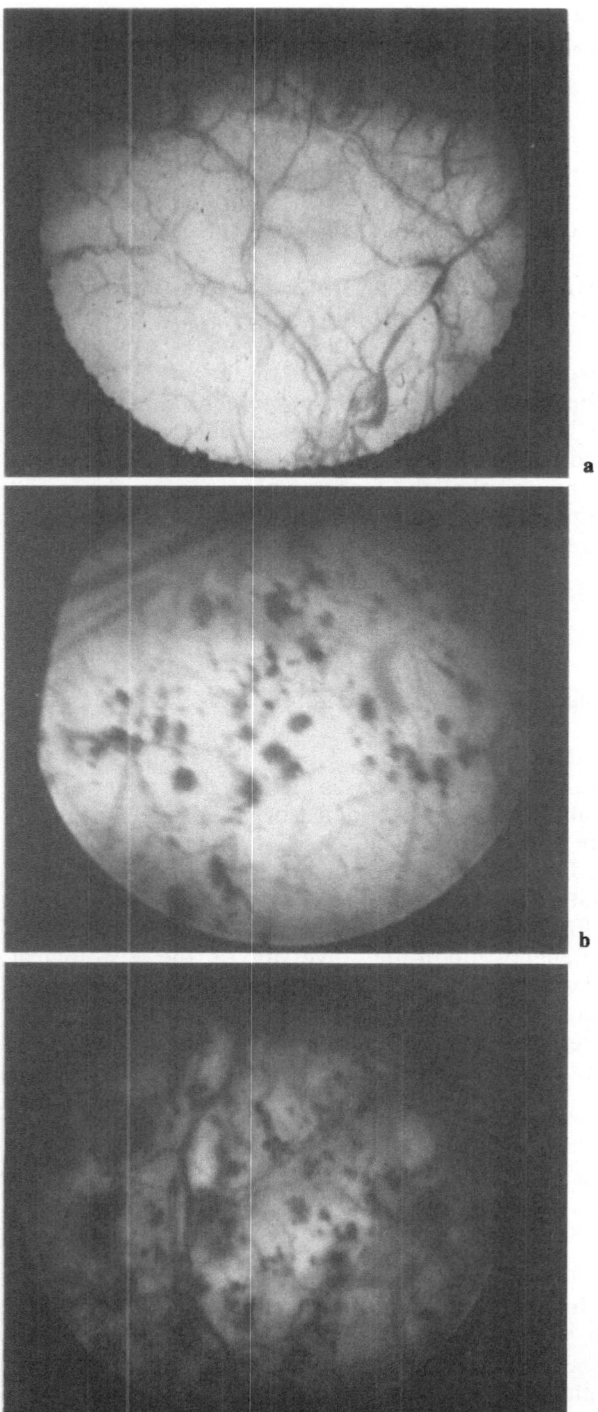

Fig. 6.7a–c. Cystoscopy in interstitial cystitis. **a** normal bladder mucosa (control patient); **b** petechial bleeding; **c** ecchymoses.

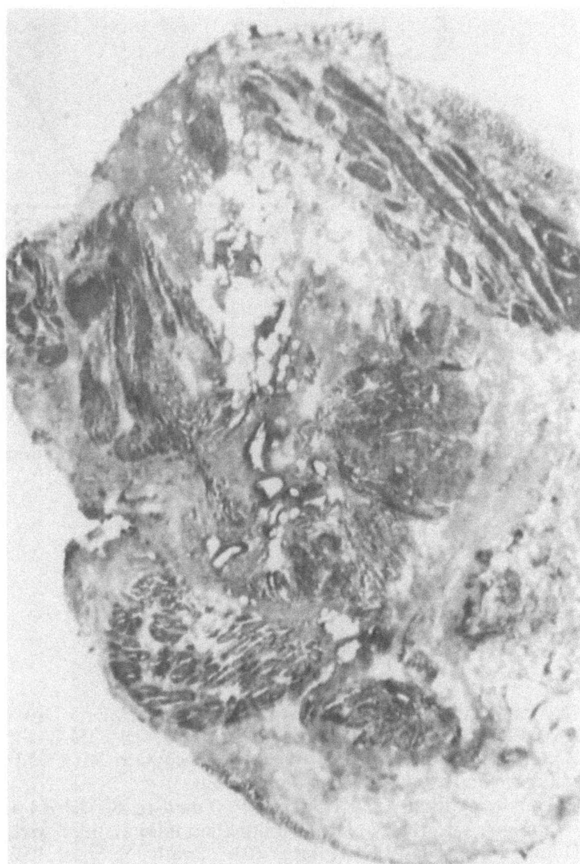

Fig. 6.8. Examples of a sufficient bladder biopsy including detrusor muscle. Stain: Masson's trichrome, ×25

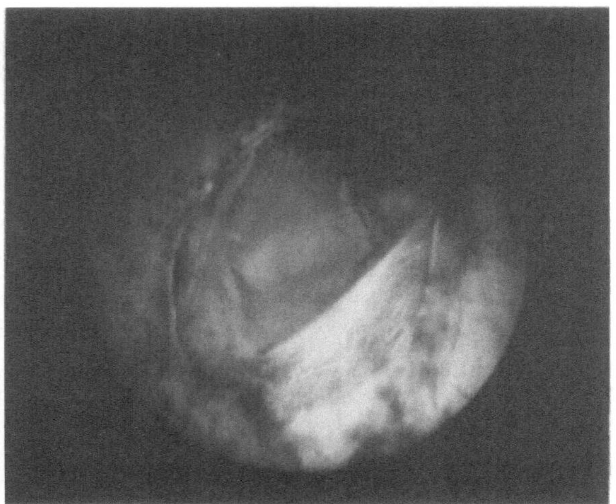

Fig. 6.9. Deep biopsy site seen cystoscopically. Catheter drainage is advised for 24 hours.

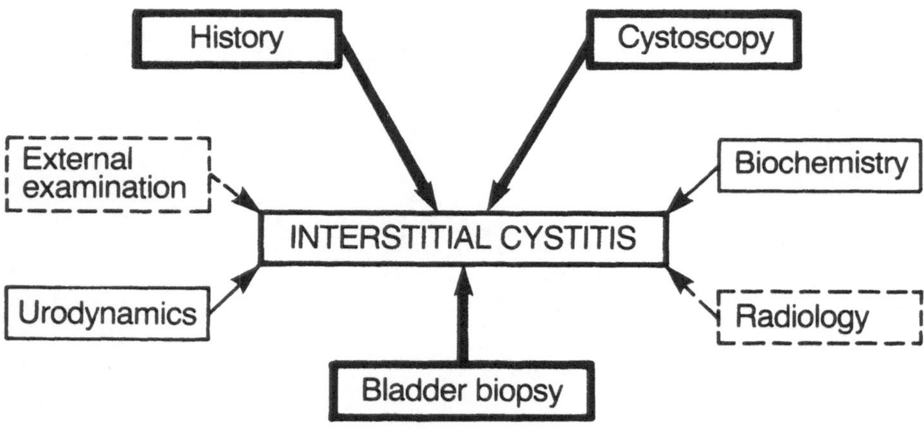

Fig. 6.10. The relative value of diagnostic methods in interstitial cystitis.

References

Badenoch AW (1971) Chronic interstitial cystitis. Br J Urol 43:718–721

BMJ Editorial (1972) Interstitial cystitis. Br Med J I:644–645

Bohne AW, Hodson JM, Rebuck JW, Reinhard RE (1962) An abnormal leukocyte response in interstitial cystitis. J Urol 88: 387–391

Collan Y, Alfthan O, Kivilaakso E, Oravisto KJ (1976) Electron microscopic and histological findings on urinary bladder epithelium in interstitial cystitis. Eur Urol 2:242–247

Dunn M, Ramsden PD, Roberts JBM, Smith JC, Smith PJB (1977) Interstitial cystitis, treated by prolonged bladder distension. Br J Urol 49:641–645

Geist RW, Antolak SJ (1970) Interstitial cystitis in children. J Urol 104:922–925

Gordon HL, Rossen RD, Hersh EM, Yium JJ (1973) Immunologic aspects of interstitial cystitis. J Urol 109:228–233

Hanash KA, Pool TL (1969) Interstitial cystitis in men. J Urol 102: 427–428

Hand JR (1949) Interstitial cystitis: Report of 223 cases (204 women and 19 men). J Urol 61:291–310

Herbst RH, Baumrucher GO, German KL (1937) Elusive ulcer (Hunner) of the bladder with an experimental study of the etiology. Am J Surg 38:152–167

Kinder CH, Smith RD (1958) Hunner's ulcer. Br J Urol 30:338–343

Lose G, Frandsen B, Højensgaard JC, Jespersen J, Astrup T (1983) Chronic interstitial cystitis: increased levels of eosinophilic cationic protein in serum and urine and an ameliorating effect of subcutaneous heparin. Scand J Urol Nephrol 17:159–161

Messing EM, Stamey TA (1978) Interstitial cystitis: Early diagnosis, pathology and treatment. Urology 12: 381–392

Oravisto KJ (1975) Epidemiology of interstitial cystitis. Ann Chir Gynaecol Fenn 64:75–77

Oravisto KJ (1980) Interstitial cystitis as an autoimmune disease: A review. Eur Urol 6:10–13

Oravisto KJ, Alfthan OS, Jokinen EJ (1970) Interstitial cystitis: Clinical and immunological findings. Scand J Urol Nephrol 4: 37–42

Silk MR (1970) Bladder antibodies in interstitial cystitis. J Urol 103: 307–309

Stamey TA (1974) Urinary infections. Williams and Wilkins, Baltimore, pp 80–123

Utz DC, Zincke H (1974) The masquerade of bladder cancer in situ as interstitial cystitis. J Urol 111:160–161

Walsh A (1978) Interstitial cystitis. In: Harrison JH, Gitles RF, Perlmutter AD, Stamey TA, Walsh PC (eds) Campbell's textbook of urology, 4th edn. Saunders, Philadelphia, pp 693–707

Chapter 7

Morphological Studies of the Bladder Wall in Interstitial Cystitis

J.S. Dixon and T. Hald

General Pathology

The available pathological evidence suggests that interstitial cystitis is associated with a pancystitis. The bladder wall is frequently thickened, the perivesical tissues are infiltrated, and there may be fixation of the bladder to surrounding structures. Microscopically there is frequent thinning of the mucosal lining, whilst in some areas the mucosa may be denuded of urothelial covering. The areas of ulceration may be covered by a layer of fibrin which sometimes contains collections of polymorphonuclear leucocytes, and squamous metaplasia is occasionally observed. The most striking changes are seen in the subepithelial connective tissue where an intense reaction occurs beneath the areas of mucosal thinning.

The lamina propria is oedematous, congested, and contains dilated capillaries and perivascular haemorrhages. Indeed, the presence of thin-walled vessels in this region may explain the tendency towards bleeding on distension of the bladder in patients with interstitial cystitis. There is a marked diffuse cellular infiltration, mainly by lymphocytes, in all layers of the bladder wall, but particularly the lamina propria (Fig. 7.1). In many cases eosinophils are observed, especially in early lesions. Mast cells are also present, particularly in relation to the blood vessels of the lamina propria.

Specific Pathology

Mast Cells

Mast cells have frequently been reported to be associated with interstitial cystitis both as a pathogenetic mechanism (Bohne et al. 1962; Simmons 1961; Smith and Dehner 1972; Kárpáti and Antal 1971, 1975) and as a pathognomonic marker (Larsen et al. 1982). Mast cells produce a number of histologically active

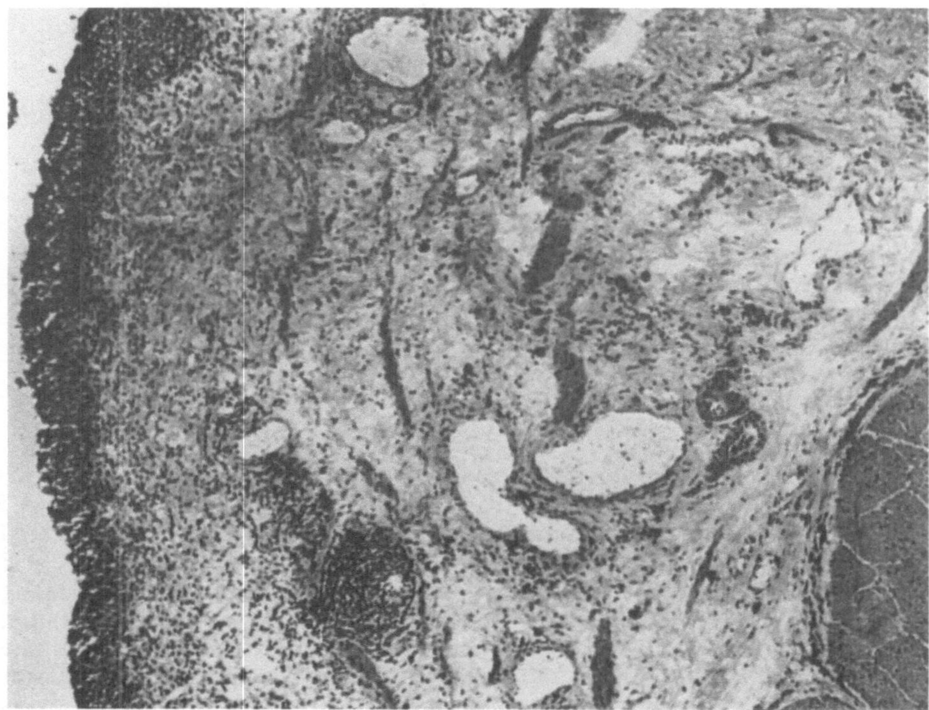

Fig. 7.1. The bladder wall in interstitial cystitis showing a diffuse infiltration of the lamina propria by lymphocytes. (×200)

compounds, of which histamine is the best described. Histamine release in tissue causes pain, hyperaemia and fibrosis, all notable features of interstitial cystitis. However, no significantly elevated histamine concentration in bladder biopsies has been found in the disease although methodological problems may be responsible for this observation (Kastrup et al. 1983).

There is no agreement as to the validity of mast cell infiltration as a diagnostic feature of interstitial cystitis (Messing and Stamey 1978). However, Larsen et al. (1982) found that 27 of a total of 32 patients with a typical history and findings on cystoscopy had elevated mast cell counts in the muscle coat (28 per mm^2) whereas the number of mast cells in the lamina propria did not differ from a control group. Furthermore, 7 out of 11 patients with a typical history but negative or equivocal cystoscopy had an elevated mast cell count in the detrusor muscle coat (Fig. 7.2). It remains to be decided whether an elevated mast cell count in the muscularis is a constant or a transient finding but longitudinal studies should eventually answer this question.

Ultrastructurally the nuclei of these mast cells frequently contain numerous very dense irregularly shaped clumps of chromatin lying adjacent to the nuclear membrane (Fig. 7.3). Such a feature has been claimed to be characteristic of degranulating mast cells (Dennison et al. 1972), although the precise aetiological factors underlying this degranulation have yet to be determined.

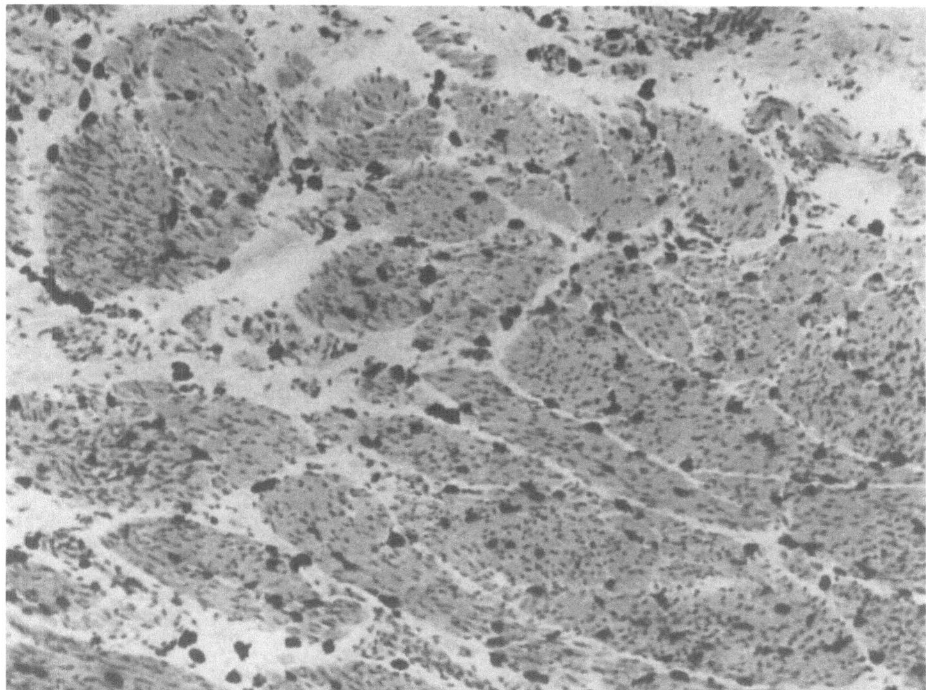

Fig. 7.2. Gross infiltration of detrusor muscle bundles by mast cells in a case of interstitial cystitis. (×1000)

Immunoglobulins

Immunofluorescence studies in interstitial cystitis have given varying results. Gordon et al. (1973) noted IgG and IgM deposits in the lamina propria and in the sarcolemma of the detrusor muscle cells. An unpublished study by Hald et al. (1983) has confirmed the existence of a number of different immunoglobulins in the bladder wall, but no definite pattern could be distinguished. Other reports (Messing and Stamey 1978) have not attached any significance to the presence of these proteins.

Submucosal Vascular Changes in Interstitial Cystitis

Fine structural studies of bladder submucosal vessel walls from patients with interstitial cystitis have demonstrated pronounced vascular injury in approximately 70% of cases (Mattila et al. 1983; Dixon 1984, unpublished observations). Severely damaged endothelial cells are commonly observed together with proliferation and multilayering of the underlying basal lamina (Fig. 7.4). The latter is sometimes disrupted by polymorphonuclear cells and the subendothelial space is relatively wide and oedematous. In approximately one third of the

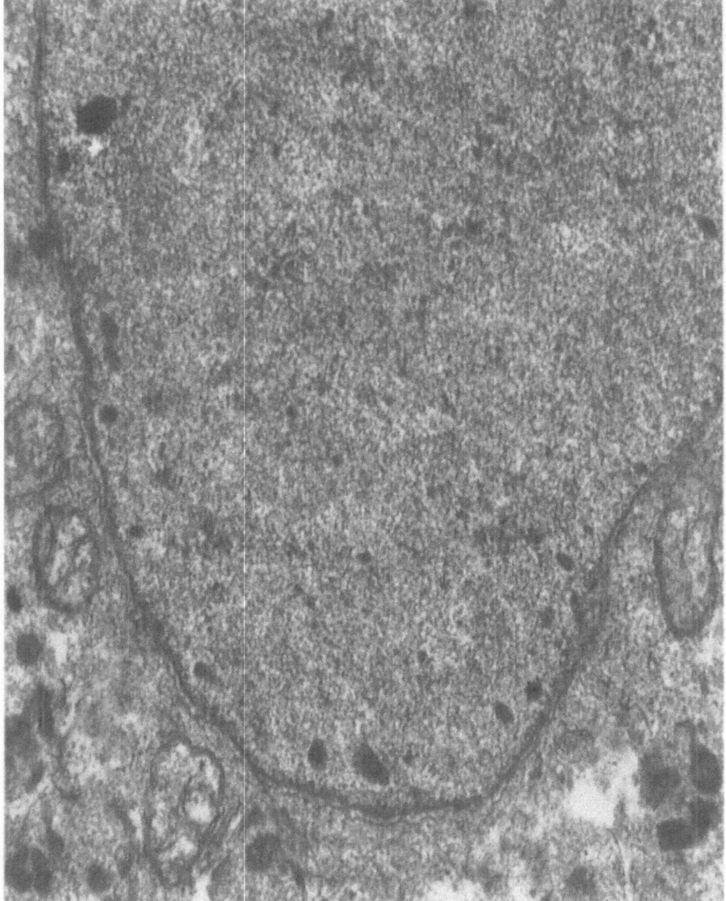

Fig. 7.3. Electron micrograph of a portion of the nucleus of a degranulating mast cell from a case of interstitial cystitis. The nucleus contains numerous irregular dense chromatin granules towards the periphery. (×35 000)

patients examined the subendothelial space contained clusters of microfibrils 10–12 nm in diameter, similar to those observed in close association with mature elastic fibres.

In these cases evidence of injury to vascular smooth muscle consists of cells which display a variety of lesions, including clumping of nuclear chromatin, swollen mitochondria, cytoplasmic vacuoles, lipid droplets and myelin figures. Seventy-five per cent of biopsy samples possessed small spherical membrane-bound vesicles associated with elastic elements occupying the intermuscular spaces of the blood vessel walls (Fig. 7.5). These vesicles are referred to as granulovesicular bodies and are believed to be associated with both regenerating and newly developing elastic elements. Mattila et al. (1983) have suggested that

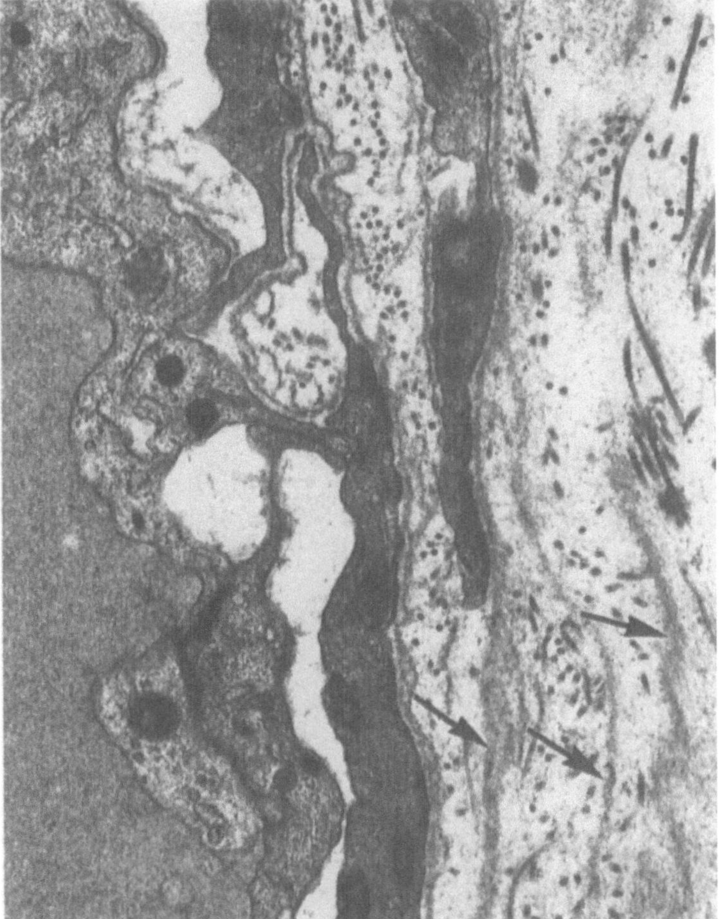

Fig. 7.4. Proliferation of basal lamina material has occurred (*arrow*) beneath the wall of a suburothelial blood vessel. (×22 500)

the newly synthesised elastic microfibrils may act as antigens in the pathogenetic process. Thus injury to the vessel walls may be due to autoantibodies or immune complexes formed within them.

Microbial infections, especially those of viral origin, have been considered as potential triggers for autoimmunisation which may lead to chronic types of vascular injury (Allison 1973; Glynn 1975). The consequent inflammation may then liberate connective tissue microfibrils, with subsequent autoimmune response. A variety of virus infections are associated with autoantibodies and are known to induce autoallergic manifestations (Allison 1973). Furthermore, it seems likely that these responses depend on genetic constitution as in other autoimmune disease (Glyn 1975).

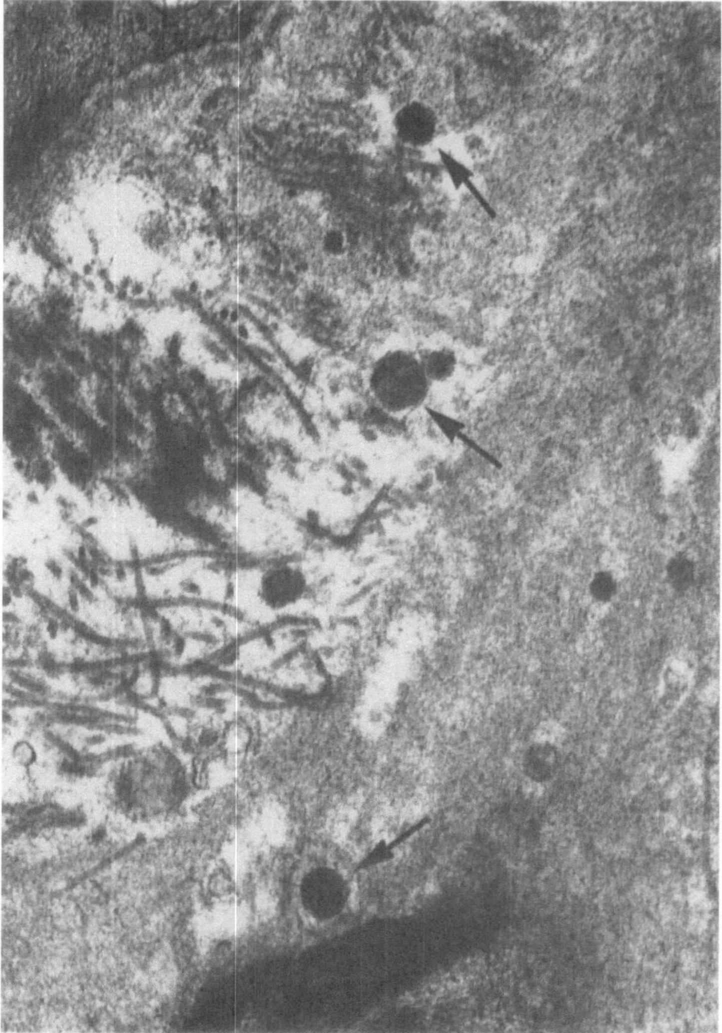

Fig. 7.5. Several membrane bound vesicles (*arrows*) occupy the intermuscular spaces of a blood vessel wall. (×35 000)

Bladder Mucosa in Interstitial Cystitis

It has been shown that the surface of the mucosa lining the urinary bladder is lined with a layer of sulphonated glycosaminoglycans (GAGs) which act as an important defence between the urothelial cells and potentially harmful substances in the urine (Parsons et al. 1977, 1980). Such a layer has been demonstrated in both the rabbit and human bladder (Fig. 7.6). Parsons et al. (1983) have proposed a theory involving a defect in this protective layer in

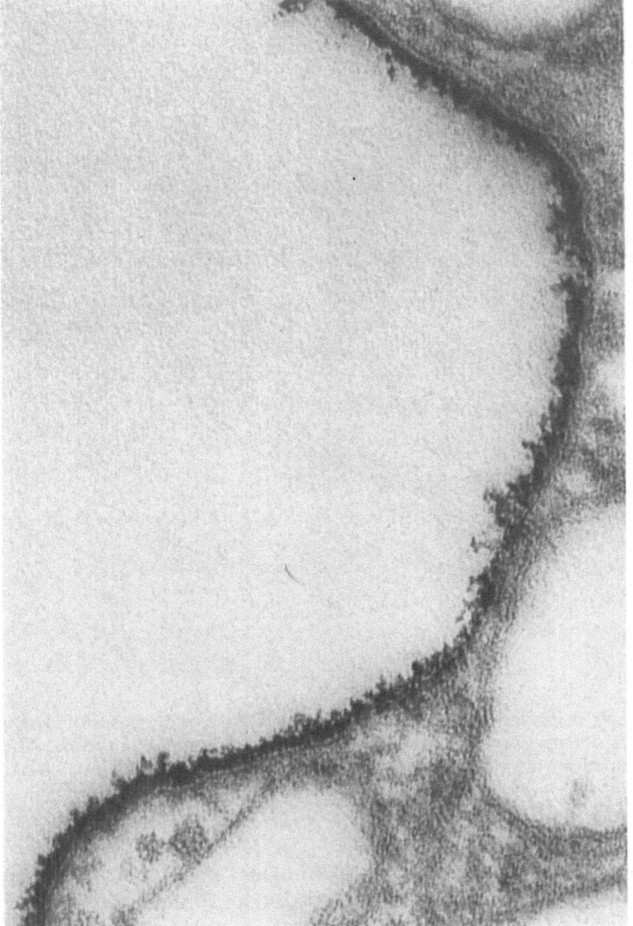

Fig. 7.6. Ruthenium red-stained glycosaminoglycans layer at the luminal surface of bladder urothelium from a case of interstitial cystitis. (×176 000)

patients with interstitial cystitis, suggesting that treatment with synthetic GAGs may be of benefit. However, a recent study by Dixon et al. (1985), using staining with ruthenium red, was unable to detect any fine structural differences between the GAG layer of interstitial cystitis patients and that from controls. Hence the hypothesis that an important pathogenetic factor in interstitial cystitis is a defective glycocalyx could not be supported.

Isotope diffusion studies, in combination with electron microscope observations of the subcellular distribution of lanthanum (Fig. 7.7), have indicated a marked increase in bladder urothelial permeability in patients with interstitial cystitis (Eldrup et al. 1983). If such observations indicate a basic epithelial defect (as was originally suggested by Gordon et al. 1973), possibly due to defective

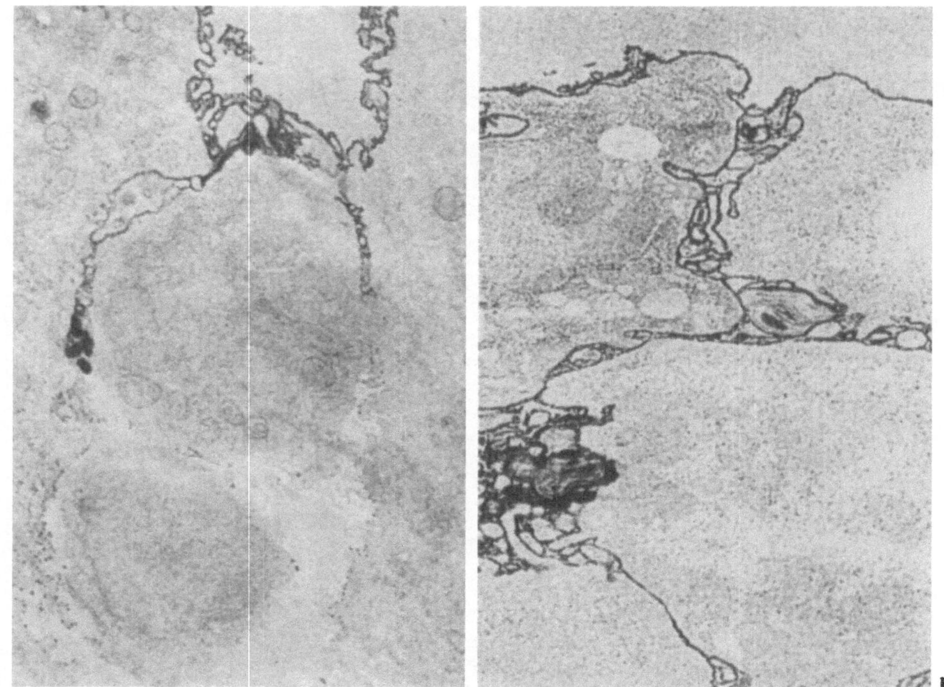

Fig. 7.7a,b. Electron microscopy using lanthanum to detect 'leaky' tight junctions. **a** Normal urothelium. The lanthanum does not penetrate beyond tight junctions. **b** Interstitial cystitis. The lanthanum leaks through tight junctions into the deeper layers of the urothelium.

urothelial tight junctions, the possibility exists that urine may leak into the bladder wall and induce a local inflammatory response. These secondary changes may explain the results of lymphocyte migration tests and the local deposition of immunoglobulins and mast cells in the wall of the bladder.

In summary, the pathogenesis of interstitial cystitis is presently unknown although a number of possible factors are listed in Table 7.1.

Table 7.1. Suggested aetiological factors in interstitial cystitis

Toxic substances from the urine
Extravesical foci of infection
Circulatory disturbances
Lymphatic obstruction
Hormonal factors
Neurogenic factors
Genetic deficiencies
Immunological disturbances

References

Allison AC (1973) (Heberden Oration, 1972) Mechanisms of tolerance and autoimmunity. Ann Rheum Dis 32:283–293

Bohne AW, Hodson JM, Rebuck JW, Reinhard RE (1962) An abnormal leukocyte response in interstitial cystitis. J Urol 88:387–391

Dennison S, Freeman R, Still WJS (1972) Nuclear changes in degranulating mast cells. Arch Pathol 93:530–531

Dixon JS, Holm-Bentzen M, Gilpin CJ, Gosling JA, Bostofte E, Hald T, Larsen S (1985) Electron microscopic investigation of the bladder urothelium and glycocalyx in patients with interstitial cystitis. J Urol (submitted for publication)

Eldrup J, Thorup J, Nielsen SL, Hald T, Hainau B (1983) Permeability and ultrastructure of human bladder epithelium. Br J Urol 55:488–492

Glynn LE (1975) Experimental models and etiology of inflammatory rheumatic diseases. Scand J Rheumatol 5:55–62

Gordon HL, Rossen RD, Hersh EM, Yium JJ (1973) Immunologic aspects of interstitial cystitis. J Urol 109:228–233

Kárpâti F, Antal A (1971) Mastocytendestruktion, eine neue therapeutische Möglichkeit bei der Behandlung der interstitiellen Cystitiden. Urologie 410:25–29

Kárpâti F, Antal A (1975) Über die lokale Blasenbehandlung von Patienten mit interstitieller Zystitis im Spiegel der Regranulation der Mastozyten. Z Urol Nephrol 68:625–631

Kastrup J, Hald T, Larsen S, Nielsen VG (1983) Histamine content and mast cell count of detrusor muscle in patients with interstitial cystitis and other types of chronic cystitis. Br J Urol 55:495–500

Larsen S, Thompson SA, Hald T, Barnard RJ, Gilpin CJ, Dixon JS, Gosling JA (1982) Mast cells in interstitial cystitis. Br J Urol 54:283–286

Mattila J, Pitkänen R, Vaalasti T, Seppänen J (1983) Fine-structural evidence for vascular injury in patients with interstitial cystitis. Virchows Arch [A] 398:347–355

Messing EM, Stamey TA (1978) Interstitial cystitis: Early diagnosis, pathology and treatment. Urology 12:381–392

Parsons CL, Greenspan C, Moore SW, Mulholland SG (1977) Role of surface mucin in primary antibacterial defence of bladder. Urology 9:48–52

Parsons CL, Stauffer C, Schmidt JD (1980) Bladder surface glycosaminoglycans: an efficient mechanism of environmental adaption. Science 208:605–607

Parsons CL, Schmidt JD, Pollen JJ (1983) Successful treatment of interstitial cystitis with sodium pentosanpolysulfate. J Urol 130:51–53

Simmons JL (1961) Interstitial cystitis: An explanation for the beneficial effect of an antihistamine. J Urol 85:149–155

Smith BH, Dehner LP (1972) Chronic ulcerating interstitial cystitis. A study of 28 cases. Arch Pathol 93:76–81

Chapter 8

Treatment of Interstitial Cystitis

T. Hald, R.J. Barnard and M. Holm-Bentzen

Introduction

The variety of therapeutic measures which have been described for the management of interstitial cystitis reflects both the uncertain aetiology of the condition as well as the difficulty in controlling the symptoms of the disorder (Table 8.1). A further problem of management relates to the individual response to therapy. Some patients, realising the chronic nature of the disorder and the limitations of available treatment, will accept that some restriction of their life-style will have to be tolerated. Other patients, however, may not be prepared to suffer any untoward frequency or discomfort, thus making the therapeutic problem that much more difficult for the clinician.

In interstitial cystitis treatment has been directed towards the bladder mucosal surface, the apparent tissue response, the decreased bladder capacity and the symptomatic relief of suprapubic pain.

Treatment

Bladder Urothelium

Treatment may be effected either by intracavity installation or by systemic administration of active compounds. A nonspecific astringent effect can be obtained by an infusion of silver nitrate as recommended by Hunner (1930), but the beneficial effects are of short duration (De Juana and Everett 1977). Electrocoagulation of mucosal lesions on the bladder surface has been employed (Franksson 1957; Greenberg et al. 1974) although this method has become less popular since the realisation that the bladder pathology is more extensive than can be identified by using the cystoscope. Heparin has been used therapeutically on the basis of its effects on the properties of the urothelium and on mast cell degranulation (Weaver et al. 1963; Kárpáti 1964). This drug is thought to induce

Table 8.1. Therapeutic principles in interstitial cystitis

Type of therapy	Primary objective of Therapy					
	Mucosa and glycocalyx	Anti-inflammatory	Immuno-suppression	Mast cells and histamine	Bladder capacity	Pain relief
Local	Silver nitrate	DMSO Chlorpactin Orgotein	Prednisone		DMSO (?) Hyal-uronidase	Subtrigonal phenol DMSO Local anaesthetics
Systemic	Heparin Elmiron	Salicylates Butazone derivatives Chloroquine	Prednisone Azathioprine	Anti-histamines Lomudal Heparin	Anti-cholin-ergics	Analgesics
Physical					Distension Electrical stimulation	Distension Electrical stimulation
Surgery	Electro-coagulation	Electro-resection			Subtotal cystectomy Entero-cysto-plasty	Cystolysis Denervation (peri-vesical or transvaginal) Sacral neur-ectomy Diversion

the formation of a hydrophilic layer on the mucosal surface which has been considered helpful in reducing mucosal permeability (see Chap. 7). Using heparin, Lose et al. (1983) noted a marked clinical improvement in patients with interstitial cystitis, which was accompanied by a considerable fall in serum and urine eosinophilic–cationic protein level. Sulphopentosan sodium (Elmiron), a drug with similar properties to heparin but with less anticoagulant activity, has recently been used with promising initial results, reducing pain and frequency in 22 of 24 patients within 4–8 weeks of treatment (Parsons et al. 1983). Further studies are awaited to confirm the benefits of this new compound.

Anti-inflammatory and Immunosuppressive Therapy

Bladder instillations using dimethylsulphoxide (DMSO) (Stewart and Shirley 1976; Ek et al. 1978), chlorpactin (Messing and Stamey 1978) and orgotein (Mayer and Schilling 1983) have previously been employed in the treatment of interstitial cystitis. The results have indicated that between 50% and 70% of the patients are temporarily relieved of their symptoms by repeated instillations. DMSO, however, is partly excreted by the lungs and its garlic odour is unpleasant for some patients. Chlorpactin has the disadvantage that a general anaesthetic is required for its use as a therapeutic agent. Symptomatic treatment with salicylates and butazone derivatives has generally proved to be disappointing, though chloroquine has been reported to provide improvement in 60%–70% of patients (Oravisto and Alfthan 1976). Immunosuppression using prednisone has been employed both topically and systematically (Johnston 1956; Kinder and Smith 1958; Badenoch 1971; Gordon et al. 1973) in the treatment of interstitial cystitis. Oravisto and Alfthan (1976) have also used azathioprine although the potentially serious side-effects of all these drugs usually preclude their use in routine clinical practice.

Antihistamine Therapy

H_1-antihistamines (Simmons 1961) are effective in only a minority of patients with interstitial cystitis and the sedative effect of the drugs is often intolerable. Lomudal (chromoglycate), which prevents the release of histamine by mast cells, has been tested by Rosin et al. (1979) and Kjer and Hald (1979). The results were disappointing, possibly due to the lack of an efficient mode of drug administration.

Therapy to Enhance Bladder Capacity

It has already been noted (p. 22) that some patients with symptom complexes suggestive of interstitial cystitis have normal bladder capacities during cystoscopic examination. Distension therapy has little part to play in the management of these cases. However, in patients with reduced bladder capacity, distension under anaesthesia is often beneficial, at least in the early stages of the disease. Occasionally simple bladder filling which occurs at the time of cystoscopy will give relief to the patient for several months (Dunn et al. 1977).

Enterocystoplasty is generally the treatment of choice in the rare patients with severely contracted bladders (Turner-Warwick 1976). The bladder wall must be resected as near to the trigone as possible and caecum, sigmoid colon or small intestine may be employed in reconstruction of the viscus. Each of these options will give essentially similar results regarding increased functional capacity. Following such operations, mucus derived from bowel epithelium will be passed in the urine and, though it rarely causes complications, the patient should be advised of this possibility.

Relief of pain is generally achieved with these procedures although some troublesome urodynamic side-effects may be encountered. Contraction waves may occur in the isolated bowel segment and occasionally may generate sufficient pressure to lead to incontinence (Fig. 8.1). Antimotility agents such as Lomotil can help in this situation. It must be emphasised that neuromuscular coordination between bladder and bowel segment does not develop, and voiding dynamics may be significantly altered following enterocystoplasty. Urine may pass both down the urethra and up into the distensible 'iatrogenic diverticulum' formed by the enteral attachment to the bladder. Such distension viewed during videocystometry may achieve alarming proportions and typically the patient may have to void several times in order to achieve an empty bladder. If enterocystoplasty fails to achieve its objectives, it may be necessary to consider urinary diversion. However, the inherent risks of long term renal failure as well as psychological or sexual problems which follow this operation will need careful consideration.

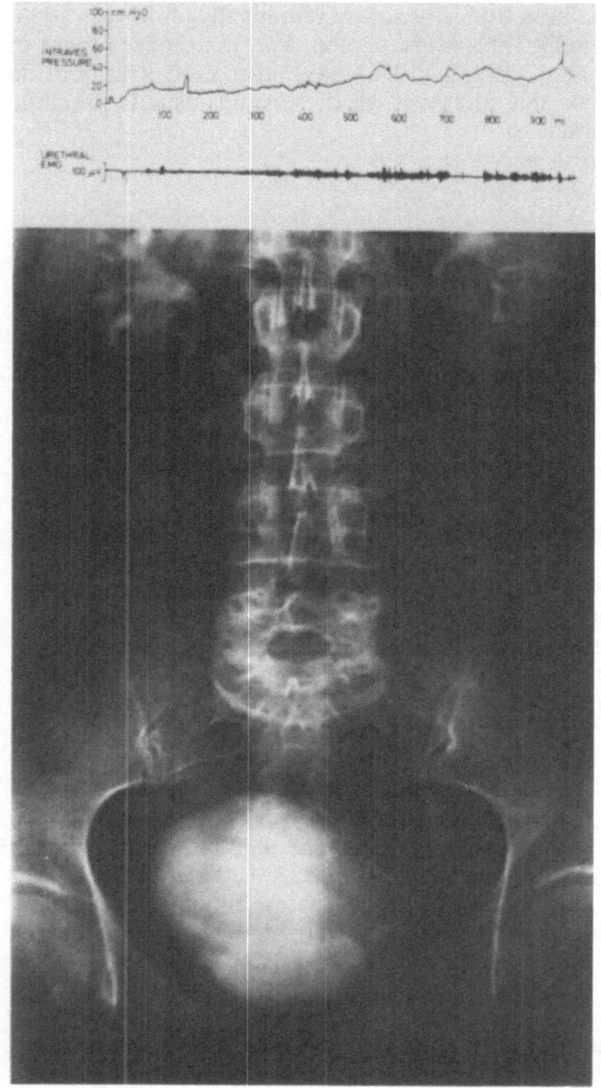

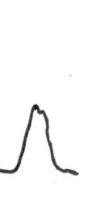

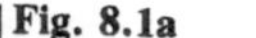
◄ Fig. 8.1a

Fig. 8.1b ▼

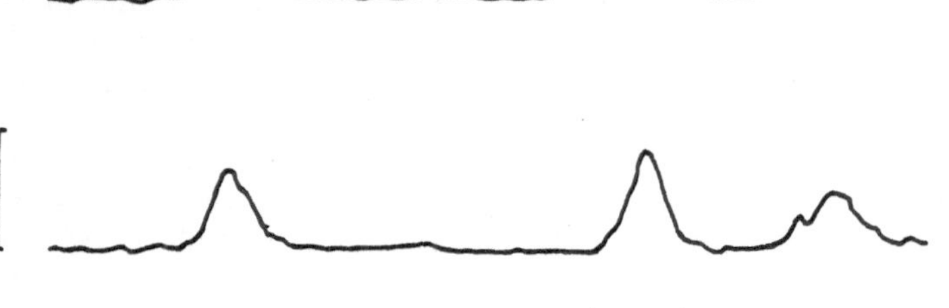

Therapy of Pain Relief

Mild analgesics are of relatively little value whilst addictive analeptic or antidepressive drugs must clearly be avoided in this chronic condition. Local anaesthetic agents administered intravesically in combination with hyaluronidase offer only temporary relief. Fall et al. (1977) have applied transvaginal electrical stimulation and report symptomatic improvement together with increased bladder capacity in a majority of cases.

Summary

Despite the large number of therapeutic options listed above the majority of patients with interstitial cystitis are managed along relatively simple and well established lines of treatment. It must be re-emphasised that most patients suspected of having the disorder usually present with relatively mild symptoms and it is rare to encounter the patient with a severely shrunken bladder and classical Hunner's ulcer.

Simple hydrostatic bladder distension under anaesthesia constitutes the initial form of therapy in the majority of patients with interstitial cystitis. Usually this procedure is effective in producing enhancement of capacity sufficient to afford relief from suprapubic pain for a reasonable period of time. Discomfort is not, however, completely abolished and the typical symptoms may be experienced if, for any reason, the patient delays micturition. Selected patients may derive additional benefit from small doses of a suitable analgesic preparation.

Instillation agents such as DMSO, despite their suitability for some cases, have not achieved widespread popularity, in part due to the garlic odour produced on the patient's breath.

It is possible that sodium sulphopentosan (Elmiron), at present undergoing a multi-centre trial, may diminish the need for cystodistension in some patients.[1]

The failure of cystodistension to alleviate symptoms in the few cases with severe disease (capacity under anaesthetic less than 100–150 ml) will lead to the patient being considered for augmentation cystoplasty. Rarely, the development of further complications in these cases may indicate the need for ileal loop diversion.

1. Editor's footnote: The result of the multi-centre trial was reported at the International Continence Society meeting in London during September 1985. Elmiron was shown not to be of benefit in the treatment of the disorder.

Fig. 8.1. **a** Spontaneous bowel contraction in a patient with interstitial cystitis and caecocystoplasty. The intravenous pyelogram shows the substantial caecal segment placed above the remains of the bladder. **b** Spontaneous bowel contractions in a 35-year-old female patient with caecocystoplasty. Pressure waves of up to 40 cm H_2O can only just be contained by the sphincter mechanism. Maximum squeeze during urethral pressure profilometry illustrated at right of trace. Vertical scale, 40 cm H_2O. Horizontal scale, 30 s. *Upper trace*, intravesical pressure. *Lower trace*, detrusor pressure. Abdominal pressure trace not illustrated.

References

Badenoch AW (1971) Chronic interstitial cystitis. Br J Urol 43:718–721

De Juana CP, Everett JC (1977) Interstitial cystitis: Experience and review of recent literature. Urology 10:325–329

Dunn M, Ramsden PD, Roberts JBM, Smith JC, Smith PJB (1977) Interstitial cystitis, treated by prolonged bladder distension. Br J Urol 49:641–645

Ek A, Engberg A, Frödin L, Jönsson G (1978) The use of dimethyl-sulfoxide (DMSO) in the treatment of interstitial cystitis. Scand J Urol Nephrol 12:129–131

Fall M, Erlandson B-E, Carlsson C-A (1977) Electrical stimulation in interstitial cystitis. Paper presented at the VIIth meeting of the International Continence Society. Portoroz, Yugoslavia

Franksson C (1957) Interstitial cystitis. A clinical study of fifty-nine cases. Acta Chir Scand 113:51–62

Gordon HL, Rossen RD, Hersh EM, Yium JJ (1973) Immunologic aspects of interstitial cystitis. J Urol 109:228–233

Greenberg E, Barnes R, Stewart S, Furnish T (1974) Transurethral resection of Hunner's ulcer. J Urol 111:764–766

Hunner GL (1930) Neurosis of the bladder. J Urol 24:567–585

Johnston JH (1956) Local hydrocortisone for Hunner's ulcer of the bladder. Br Med J II:698–699

Kárpáti F (1964) Behandlung des Ulcus simplex vesicae urinariae (Hunnersches Geschwür) mit Heparin. Urol Nephrol 57:895–898

Kinder CH, Smith RD (1958) Hunner's ulcer. Br J Urol 30:338–343

Kjer JJ, Hald T (1979) Oral sodium cromoglicate (Lomudal) in the treatment of interstitial cystitis. Paper presented to the Danish Surgical Society, annual meeting, Copenhagen, Denmark

Lose G, Frandsen B, Højensgaard JC, Jespersen J, Astrup T (1983) Chronic interstitial cystitis: increased levels of eosinophilic cationic protein in serum and urine and an ameliorating effect of subcutaneous heparin. Scand J Urol Nephrol 17:159–161

Mayer P, Schilling A (1983) Medikamentöse Rehabilitation der interstitiellen Cystitis mit Orgotein. Paper presented at the 25th Congress of the North German Urological Association. Denmark

Messing EM, Stamey TA (1978) Interstitial cystitis, early diagnosis, pathology and treatment. Urology 12:381–392

Oravisto KJ, Alfthan OS (1976) Treatment of interstitial cystitis with immunosuppression and chloroquine derivatives. Eur Urol 2:82–84

Parsons CL, Schmidt JD, Pollen JJ (1983) Successful treatment of interstitial cystitis with sodium pentosanpolysulfate. J Urol 130:51–53

Rosin RD, Griffiths T, Sofras F, James DCO, Edwards L (1979) Interstitial cystitis. Br J Urol 51:524–527

Simmons JL (1961) Interstitial cystitis: An explanation for the beneficial effect of an antihistamine. J Urol 85:149–155

Stewart BH, Shirley SW (1976) Further experience with intravesical dimethyl sulfoxide in the treatment of interstitial cystitis. J Urol 116:36–38

Turner-Warwick R (1976) Cystoplasty. In: Blandy J (ed) Urology. Blackwells, Oxford, pp 840–856

Weaver RG, Dougherty TF, Natoli CA (1963) Recent concepts in interstitial cystitis. J Urol 89:377–383

Section 3

The Urethral Syndrome

Chapter 9

Historical Review—Confusions in Definition

C.A.C. Charlton

"When I use a word", Humpty Dumpty said in a rather scornful tone, "it means just what I choose it to mean,—neither more nor less."

Lewis Carroll (1871)

This quotation from *Alice Through the Looking Glass* nicely illustrates one of several major problems which face those interested in the diagnosis and treatment of symptom complexes which apparently arise from the female urinary tract. Before 1940 terms such as neuralgia of the bladder, granular urethritis, rheumatic urethritis, cystitis trigoni and cystitis colli were in common use for the description of lower tract symptoms associated with clear urine (Ormond 1935). Equally broad was the dictum of the distinguished American physician Richard Cabot as paraphrased by Folsom: "Any pain within two feet of the female urethra for which one cannot find an adequate explanation, should be suspected of coming from the female urethra." (Folsom 1945)

The term 'urethral syndrome' was first mentioned in a clinico-pathological study of the female urethra reported in 1949 by Powell and Powell. Since that time the syndrome has been widely recognised but absence of definitive criteria has resulted in both inconsistency and confusion in the literature relating to the disorder. The urethral syndrome is first and foremost a diagnosis of exclusion. The clinician must seek to exclude by all possible means any pathological process that might conceivably give rise to symptoms centred upon the lower urinary tract. Previous pelvic trauma or radiation injury resulting from treatment of rectal, uterine or bladder neoplasia may explain the symptom complex, as may the chemical cystitis which occasionally follows systemic chemotherapy (e.g. cyclophosphamide) for myeloproliferative disease. Carcinoma in situ and subepithelial carcinoma of the bladder are conditions which also require exclusion by appropriate techniques. Gynaecological abnormalities may trap the unwary who may assign the syndrome label before a thorough examination under anaesthetic has been undertaken. Uterine malignancy, fibroids or ovarian cyst (Davidson and Matheson 1964) can on occasion present with urethral discomfort, urgency and frequent desire to void.

The exclusion of extraneous disease process leads to a consideration of the exact role played by urinary and genital tract infection in the spectrum of symptom complexes arising from the female lower urinary tract. The urethral syndrome occupies part of this spectrum but needs to be clearly distinguished from the infectious and inflammatory disorders by precise definitive criteria, agreed and accepted by all physicians concerned in the management of the patient. The problems of terminology which arise under these circumstances are covered elsewhere (p. 25) and the microbiology of the female urethra is fully described on p. 85.

The urethral syndrome is defined using a combination of clinical symptoms and a microbiological assessment of fractional urine samples. Frequency and abacteriuria are essential criteria and whilst the most typical examples of the syndrome do not have white blood cells in their urine, the presence of leucocytes does not exclude the diagnosis. Abacteriuria means organisms are not recovered in any concentration from either initial (VB1) or midstream (VB2) urine samples. Patients with 'non-significant' bacteriuria (less than 10^5 per ml) do not qualify for inclusion into the syndrome (see p. 23). The tubercle bacillus and carbon dioxide-dependent organisms will of course be excluded by appropriate bacterial culture. Specific techniques for the isolation of *Chlamydia trachomatis* are required to identify this organism, which was noted to be associated with the urethral syndrome (though not always isolated from the urethra) in 10 of 16 pyuric patients studied by Stamm et al. (1980).

These observations refer to 'single swab' examinations; the results obtained after examination of the patient on a single occasion. It is important to appreciate that with time significant variations occur in the microbiology of the female lower urinary tract. Abacteriuric patients conforming to the syndrome as defined above were followed for several months by O'Grady and co-workers (1973) and found to fall into two distinct groups. Patients in whom fractional urine (VB2) samples demonstrated persistent white blood cells within urine (greater than 20 cu mm) developed bacteriuria periodically whilst at other times the urine remained sterile. Hence in these patients the diagnosis of the urethral syndrome depended to a large extent on the timing of the bacteriological investigation. The second group of patients, in whom the urine remained acellular for many months, were considered to have a separate condition from the 'between infections' patients (O'Grady et al. 1973). Longitudinal follow-up is also necessary to assess the fluctuations in introital colonisation by pathogenic coliform organisms. Studies on asymptomatic controls have shown that enterobacteria are carried at the introitus in approximately 23% of normal women (O'Grady et al. 1970), though the absolute numbers of organisms are generally less than those isolated in groups of symptomatic patients (Stamey and Sexton 1975). Introital coliforms were recovered during follow-up in 67% of patients with recurrent lower urinary tract symptoms and these persistent carriers suffered most frequently from urinary tract infection (O'Grady et al. 1970), thus confirming previous studies linking carriage rate to infection (Cox et al. 1968). Similar observations were made by Stamey and Sexton (1975), who repeatedly swabbed the introitus of patients with histories of recurrent lower urinary tract infection *between* bacteriuric episodes, and found an *E. coli* carrier rate of 54%. No antibiotics were permitted in this study except during bacteriuric periods when swabs were not taken. It was noted, however, that 43% of cultures from patients were free of gram-negative organisms (Stamey and Sexton 1975).

These studies emphasise the difficulties encountered when attempting to interpret microbiological findings in patients who are seen on single visits to the clinic. The intermittent nature of bacteriuria, the ebb and flow of introital colonisation and the long term remission seen after successful antimicrobial therapy (Kunin 1970) ensure that a confident diagnosis of the urethral syndrome will not be made until a considerable number of observations and investigations have been made over an extended period of time.

Charlton et al. (1973) sought to investigate the role of the urethra in the urethral syndrome. Studies of washout or initial (VBI) urine samples did not, however, show convincing or consistent results as regards the relationship of either white blood cells or organisms with the patient's symptoms. Urethral mucosal smears taken simultaneously with introital swabs were submitted to cytological examination but inflammatory urethral changes were identified in only 25% of those patients in whom enterobacteria were recovered from the adjacent introital area. It was considered that the presence of symptoms in patients with apparently normal urethras might in part be explained by the use of vaginal deodorants, foams, gels, bubble baths, or contact with diaphragms or sheaths used for contraception. The largely negative results obtained from this investigation prompted the description of these patients as suffering from the 'non-urethral syndrome', a term reflecting the condition as seen from the medical rather than the patient's point of view.

Patients with symptoms of frequency and dysuria in association with negative urinalysis of fractional urine samples and sterile urine cultures on repeated testing constitute the 'hard core' of the urethral syndrome. Additionally, a number of symptomatic but abacteriuric patients with white blood cells in their urine (persistent or intermittent) will eventually warrant classification under the same heading (Stamm et al. 1980). However, the response to antibiotic therapy in the latter patients emphasises possible aetiological differences between the two groups (Stamm et al. 1981).

References

Charlton CAC, Cattell WR, Canti G, Grottick J, O'Grady FW (1973) The non-urethral syndrome. In: Brumfitt W, Asscher AW (eds) Urinary tract infection. Oxford University Press, Oxford, pp 173–177

Cox CE, Lacey SS, Hinman F Jr (1968) The urethra and its relationship to urinary tract infection. II. The urethral flora of the female with recurrent urinary infection. J Urol 99:632

Davidson AI, Matheson NA (1964) Ovarian cysts and urinary symptoms. Br J Surg 51:908–910

Everett HS (1941) Urology in the female. Am J Surg 52:521–659

Folsom AI, O'Brien HA (1945) The female urethra. JAMA 128:408–414

Kunin CM (1970) The natural history of recurrent bacteriuria in school-girls. N Engl J Med 282:1441

O'Grady FW, Richards B, McSherry MA, O'Farrell SM, Cattell WR (1970) Introital enterobacteria, urinary infection and the urethral syndrome. Lancet II:1208–1210

O'Grady FW, Charlton CAC, Kelsey-Fry I, McSherry A, Cattell WR (1973) Natural history of intractable 'cystitis' in women referred to a special clinic. In: Brumfitt W, Asscher AW (eds.) Urinary tract infection. Oxford University Press, Oxford, pp 81–91

Ormond JK (1935) Non-purulent urethritis in women. J Urol 33:483–497

Powell NB, Powell EB (1949) The female urethra: A clinico-pathological study. J Urol 61:557

Stamey TA, Sexton CC (1975) The role of vaginal colonization and enterobacteriaceae in recurrent urinary infections. J Urol 113:214–217

Stamm WE, Wagner KF, Amsel R, Alexander ER, Turck M, Counts GW, Holmes KK (1980) Causes of the acute urethral syndrome in women. N Engl J Med 303:409–415

Stamm WE, Running K, McKevitt M, Counts GW, Turck M, Holmes KK (1981) Treatment of the acute urethral syndrome. N Engl J Med 304:956–958

Chapter 10

Microbiology of the Female Urethra and Adjacent Areas

S.J. Richmond

Introduction

The diagnosis of the urethral syndrome is a diagnosis of exclusion, made in women who have classical symptoms of urinary tract infection, but in whom no infection is found when freshly voided midstream urine (MSU; also known as VB2) is examined by conventional bacteriological techniques. However, some women who appear 'uninfected' by standard tests nevertheless have significant numbers of polymorphonuclear cells in their urine, and recent studies have indicated that more sophisticated microbiological investigation of both urine and urethra sometimes reveals infections in these pyuric women which otherwise go unrecognised. This suggests that a more critical microbiological appraisal of patients with the apparent urethral syndrome is needed, in order to define accurately the true syndrome; that is, patients with frequency and occasional dysuria in the absence of any infection of the upper or lower urinary tract.

It must be emphasised, however, that the relative importance of microbes in the aetiology of the syndrome is likely to vary considerably depending on the population of patients under investigation. For instance, approximately half the women who present for primary medical care with dysuria and frequency do not have infected urine (organisms $>10^5$ per ml, Mond et al. 1965), but only a small proportion of these women who suffer from the 'acute urethral syndrome' as defined by Stamm et al. (1980) will develop the long-standing problems which commonly warrant referral to urodynamic clinics. The latter patients, who have persistent or frequently recurring symptoms, have usually already been unsuccessfully treated with several courses of antibiotics before referral to specialist clinics. The role of microbes in the aetiology of the symptom complex in these two groups of women will probably be quite different. Similarly, the incidence and possible causal role of sexually transmitted organisms will vary considerably, and depend on the sexual exposure of the women studied.

In this chapter the common microbes—both commensals and pathogens — which frequently colonise the different epithelial surfaces in the vicinity of the urethra and which may infect the urethra itself will be reviewed. Infections of the lower urinary tract that are liable to be missed on routine tests, and which may therefore present as the urethral syndrome, are also considered.

Microbiology of the Female Lower Genito-urinary Tract

Table 10.1 lists the microbes which are commonly found in the neighbourhood of the urethra. Both commensals and potential pathogens in this area vary considerably from one epithelial surface to another. The bladder, and probably also the endocervical canal, are normally sterile, whereas the skin and the vagina support two quite different populations of commensal organisms; moreover the flora of the vagina varies considerably with changes in vaginal pH. When the pH is raised the lactobacilli which predominate under acid conditions are replaced by the bacteroides species, by aerophilic, microaerophilic and anaerobic streptococci, and by *Gardnerella vaginalis*. The pathogenicity of the latter organism is uncertain (Lancet 1978), since it probably exploits rather than causes the abnormal vaginal environment. Since the vaginitis supposedly caused by *G. vaginalis* responds to metronidazole (as do the anaerobes which are also present) the exact role of the organism in vaginitis is difficult to determine. The skin in the genital area, in addition to normal commensals such as *Staphylococcus epidermidis*, is frequently contaminated with enterobacteria. Colonisation of the introitus with *Escherichia coli* is common both in asymptomatic women and in those with the urethral syndrome (O'Grady et al. 1970). These organisms, when they gain access to and multiply in the bladder, account for about 85% of urinary tract infections which occur in domiciliary practice. *Proteus mirabilis* and *Staph. epidermidis* also cause a significant number of infections, particularly in young sexually active women. All three species cause spontaneous urinary tract infection, whereas infection of the bladder with other organisms (e.g. *Strep. faecalis*, *Klebsiella*, *Pseudomonas* and other enterobacteria) is generally the consequence of medical or surgical intervention, particularly instrumentation of the urethra.

Table 10.1. Micro-organisms found in female lower genito-urinary tract

Site	Normal flora	Pathogens
Vulva and perineum (keratinised stratified squamous epithelium)	*Staph. epidermidis* and other skin commensals Enterobacteria	*Staph. aureus, Strep. pyogenes* Herpes simplex virus[a] Genital wart virus[a]
Bladder (transitional epithelium)	Sterile	*E. coli*[b], *Proteus mirabilis*[b], *Staph. epidermidis*[b], *Klebsiella*[c], *Strep. faecalis*[c] and other enterobacteria[c]
Vagina and vaginal cervix (mucosal stratified squamous epithelium)	*Lactobacilli*[d], genital mycoplasma[d], *Bacteroides* sp[e], aerobic and anaerobic streptococci[e], genital mycoplasma[e], *Gardnerella vaginalis*[e]	*Candida albicans, Trichomonas vaginalis*[a] Herpes simplex virus[a]
Endocervix (columnar epithelium)	Sterile or vaginal commensals	*Neisseria gonorrhoeae*[a], *Chlamydia trachomatis*[a]

[a] Sexually transmitted
[b] Cause spontaneous urinary tract infections
[c] Cause urinary tract infection secondary to instrumentation
[d] Occur under conditions of normal pH
[e] Occur when pH is raised

Table 10.2. Micro-organisms found in female urethra

Site	Normal flora	Pathogens
Meatus and distal urethra (mucosal stratified squamous epithelium)	Perineal and vaginal commensals	Herpes simplex virus[a]
Proximal urethra (columnar and transitional epithelium)	Sterile or introital commensals	*Neisseria gonorrhoeae*[a] *Chlamydia trachomatis*[a]

[a] Sexually transmitted

The majority of the pathogens of the cervix, vagina and skin in the genital area (viz. *Neisseria gonorrhoeae, Trichomonas vaginalis, Chlamydia trachomatis*, and herpes simplex and genital wart viruses) are sexually transmitted. These infections are therefore most common in young women with multiple sex partners.

The microbiology of the urethra (Table 10.2), despite its easy access, is difficult to investigate with accuracy, since samples frequently contain contaminants from adjacent areas. The squamous epithelium of the meatus and distal part of the urethra is normally colonised by vaginal and perineal commensals. In contrast, the proximal part, which is lined by columnar and transitional epithelial cells, may often be sterile (Obrink et al. 1979). The urethral environment favours organisms which either have the ability to adhere firmly to the mucosal cells (e.g. gonococci and certain strains of *E. coli*), or which can grow within the cells of the urothelium (e.g. herpes simplex virus and *C. trachomatis*). It is also possible that a reservoir of infection is established in the para-urethral glands, from which reinfection of the urethral may occur. Because of sampling problems, little is known of the microbiology of these glands, but *N. gonorrhoeae* may well establish persistent infection in these structures which are lined by columnar epithelium. The pathogens of the vagina (*Candida albicans* and *T. vaginalis*) do not invade the female urethra, and the suggestion that fastidious lactobacilli cause the urethral syndrome (Maskell et al. 1979) has subsequently been refuted (Brumfitt et al. 1981). There is also no evidence that genital mycoplasmas (*Mycoplasma hominis* and *Ureaplasma urealyticum*), which frequently colonise the vagina of sexually active women, are involved in the syndrome (Stamm et al. 1980). Endocervical pathogens, notably *N. gonorrhoeae* and *C. trachomatis*, can frequently be recovered from the urethra of women with endocervical infections; this is probably a reflection of the fact that columnar epithelial cells similar to those of the endocervix, and therefore susceptible to invasion by the same microbes, occur within the urethra. The possible role of chlamydia and gonococci in the urethral syndrome is discussed below.

The Role of Potential Bladder Pathogens in the Urethral Syndrome

The role of these organisms, particularly *E. coli*, has recently been the subject of debate (Lancet 1982). In order to reach the bladder, these microbes must pass up the urethra, and probably actually colonise the urothelium in the process. Despite this, there is little evidence at present to suggest that growth of *E. coli* in the urethra causes urinary tract symptoms. The argument rather hinges on whether cystitis due to these organisms is missed because of the insensitive diagnostic criteria which are applied. Recovery of less than 10^5 organisms per ml from MSU when there has been no recent antibiotic treatment is generally regarded as insignificant. This diagnostic guideline was originally put forward by Kass (1956) to distinguish genuine bacteriuria from contaminants in the diagnosis of asymptomatic pyelonephritis, but it has subsequently been generally accepted for the diagnosis of cystitis. However, it has long been recognised that marked frequency may produce lower counts, and recent work has thrown further doubts on the reliability of quantitative analysis of MSU for the diagnosis of cystitis (Stamm et al. 1980, 1982). These workers subjected young female college students with acute dysuria and frequency to detailed microbiological investigation, and they compared results of culture of voided urine with culture of bladder urine (obtained by suprapubic aspiration or by catheterisation). They isolated *E. coli* from the bladder urine in 98 of 187 symptomatic women; all 98 patients were pyuric, but only 50% had 'significant bacteriuria' in MSU specimens (Stamm et al. 1982). Moreover some patients whose bladder urine was infected had less than 10^3 organisms per ml of voided urine. These workers argue that a bacteriuria of 10^5 per ml or more is an insensitive diagnostic test for symptomatic lower urinary tract infections.

If this work is confirmed a proportion of women diagnosed as suffering from the urethral syndrome may actually have unrecognised cystitis. This might explain why some women with the syndrome soon develop bacteriologically confirmed cystitis if they are not treated (O'Grady et al. 1970). More critical examination of MSU specimens, and reappraisal of the diagnostic criteria used for lower urinary tract infection, is therefore indicated.

The Role of Sexually Transmitted Organisms in the Urethral Syndrome

Both *N. gonorrhoea* and *C. trachomatis* are sexually transmitted organisms which may infect the female urethra as well as the endocervix. However, at both these sites these infections are very frequently asymptomatic, and the majority of women harbouring these organisms who are identified in sexually transmitted disease clinics do not complain of dysuria or frequency. Nevertheless, some recent reports suggest that *C. trachomatis* (which is an obligate intracellular bacterium and therefore not recognised by standard bacteriological techniques) may occasionally present as the urethral syndrome. For example, *C. trachomatis* infections were identified in 11 of 59 symptomatic patients (10 of whom had pyuria), compared with 3 of 66 asymptomatic control women (Stamm et al. 1980). However, chlamydia were not always recovered from the urethra itself. A recent controlled study has revealed a surprisingly high level of chlamydia urethral infection (59%) in women with the syndrome (Weil et al. 1981). An uncontrolled study of the urethral syndrome in women who attended a sexually transmitted disease clinic also identified a number of chlamydial and gonococcal infections (Panja 1983). Further controlled studies are needed both to confirm this association between sexually transmitted organisms and the syndrome, and also to demonstrate that this association is causal, rather than merely a reflection of a promiscuous life-style.

Conclusions

There are several problems associated with microbiological investigations of the urethral syndrome. It is difficult to obtain samples from the urethra which are not contaminated from adjacent areas. Differences in study populations may yield quite different results, and there are conflicting views about the significance of low ($<10^5$) numbers of bacteria in voided urine. Recent work suggests that a proportion of pyuric women with the syndrome may actually have lower urinary tract infections (viz. cystitis, or sexually transmitted infections of the urethra), which are unrecognised by standard bacteriological tests. Efforts should be made to identify these infected patients, and to distinguish them from other patients with the urethral syndrome, since in the latter group the syndrome is likely to have a quite different aetiology.

Acknowledgement. I am grateful to Professor A. Percival for his help in the preparation of this manuscript.

References

Brumfitt W, Hamilton-Miller JMT, Ludlam H, Gooding A (1981) Lactobacilli do not cause frequency and dysuria syndrome. Lancet II:393–395

Kass EH, Finland M (1956) Asymptomatic infections of the urinary tract. Trans Assoc Am Physicians 69:56–64

Lancet (1978) *Haemophilus vaginalis* in nonspecific vaginitis. Lancet II:459–460

Lancet (1982) Can kasstigation beat the truth out of the urethral syndrome? Lancet II:694–695

Maskell R, Pead L, Allen J (1979) The puzzle of "urethral syndrome": a possible answer? Lancet I:1058–1059

Mond NC, Percival A, Williams JD, Brumfitt W (1965) Presentation, diagnosis and treatment of urinary-tract infections in general practice. Lancet I:514–516

Obrink A, Bunne G, Hedlund P-O (1979) Cultures from different parts of the urethra in female urethral syndrome. Urol Int 34:70–75

O'Grady FW, Richards B, McSherry MA, O'Farrell SM, Cattell WR (1970) Introital enterobacteria, urinary infection and the urethral syndrome. Lancet II:1208–1210

Panja SK (1983) Urethral syndrome in women attending a clinic for sexually transmitted diseases. Br J Vener Dis 59:179–181

Stamm WE, Wagner KF, Amsel R, Alexander ER, Turck M, Counts GW, Holmes KK (1980) Causes of the acute urethral syndrome in women. N Engl J Med 303: 409–415

Stamm WE, Counts GW, Running KR, Fihn S, Turck M, Holmes KK (1982) Diagnosis of coliform infection in acutely dysuric women. N Engl J Med 307:463–468

Weil A, Gandenz R, Burgener L, Schultz B (1981) Isolation of *Chlamydia trachomatis* from women with the urethral syndrome. Arch Gynecol 230:329–333

Chapter 11

Urethral Syndrome—Clinical Features

N.J.R. George

Definition of Urethral Syndrome

The clinical symptom complex herein described refers to female patients who have been thoroughly screened to exclude vesical motor dysfunction (bladder instability) as well as both generalised (e.g. systemic lupus erythematosus) and local (e.g. trauma, tumour, irradiation injury or urinary infection) disease.

The essential definition of the female urethral syndrome refers to the symptoms of frequency and occasional dysuria in the absence of bacteriuria and pyuria in both initial (VB1) and midstream (VB2) urine when analysis is made on several separate occasions. The significance of positive introital culture is discussed below. Although abacteriuria is a prerequisite for the diagnosis, some patients exhibit pyuria for which no cause can be found and these patients may also be described as suffering from the urethral syndrome.

Incidence

Women suffering from symptoms related to the lower urinary tract may represent up to one-third of new patient referrals seen in the urological clinic (Smith 1979). A specific diagnosis will eventually be made in the majority of these women but there will remain a small but significant number who, by a process of elimination, conform to the urethral syndrome as defined above. The exact incidence is difficult to determine from the literature largely because of the variable diagnostic criteria used by different groups of workers.

The syndrome probably affects women of all ages though it is best expressed and studied in young women before other disorders (e.g. stress incontinence) add further to the patient's symptoms. Reports that the syndrome may occur in children (Kaplan et al. 1980) should be interpreted with caution. The possibility of anatomical abnormality (Meadow et al. 1969) and the observation that in prepubertal girls symptoms rarely arise in the absence of bacteriuria (BMJ 1977) should be borne in mind.

History

Although many patients describe an insidious onset to their symptoms some recognise that an attack of bacterial cystitis coincides with the start of the disorder. This initial or 'priming' infection is often severe, involving haematuria as well as dysuria, and though it usually resolves rapidly with antibiotics, the urethral symptoms eventually return after a variable interval despite the presence of sterile urine. However, it is recognised that although the severity of the initial attack usually leads to prompt and thorough urinalysis, many subsequent visits to the general practitioner tend to be poorly investigated and objective evidence of recurrent infection is often lacking (Mabry et al. 1981).

The symptom complex pursues a cyclical pattern in some patients who described 'attacks' which last for a variable time followed by periods of remission which may extend from a few days to several months. The factors responsible for the exacerbation of symptoms remain unclear. In some patients acid drinks (e.g. lime juice) are blamed whilst others avoid caffeine or spicy foods. Some patients relate their symptoms to menstruation or the premenstrual period, describing non-specific sensations of lower abdominal 'distension.' In the majority, however, no specific cause can be identified for the onset of symptoms.

Frequency by day is the primary complaint of most patients who describe a constant urethral 'niggle' or 'nag' which is only temporarily relieved by voiding (sensory urgency). On occasion, however, voiding may be postponed for several hours if the patient so desires (O'Boyle and Parsons 1979), thus clearly distinguishing the group from those with motor urgency who are usually unable to postpone micturition. Nocturia, even during an 'attack', is usually of mild degree (Klevmark 1981; Powell and Yeates 1982) and certainly never reaches the levels experienced by patients with interstitial cystitis (see p. 50).

Micturition is typically rather slow and hesitant (Webster 1975; O'Boyle and Parsons 1979; Jarvis 1982; Smith et al. 1981). The reduced flow rate is largely responsible for the erroneous diagnosis of 'obstruction' in these patients, the assumption being that low flow infers raised detrusor pressure during micturition. Urodynamic studies have shown this explanation to be incorrect (see p. 109).

Urethral discomfort *during voiding* is usually not severe when compared with the pain experienced during bacterial cysto-urethritis. However, if bladder overfilling occurs acute discomfort is sometimes felt at the commencement of the stream. Suprapubic ache is a common cause for complaint, which may also be exacerbated by delaying micturition. Occasionally loin pain is experienced though investigations almost invariably reveal normal renal and ureteric function. The difficulty that may be experienced in distinguishing some patients with suprapubic discomfort from atypical cases of interstitial cystitis has been discussed on p. 22.

Urethral Hypersensitivity and Allied Conditions

Urethral Hypersensitivity and Incontinence

The diagnosis of bladder instability on the basis of the history alone is notoriously difficult in female patients. Indeed a correct prediction of this dysfunction by an expert clinician is achieved in less than 50% of cases (Shepherd et al. 1982). Urodynamic investigation is therefore essential to exclude those patients whose 'urethral' symptoms are due to unstable bladder contractions, and hence urge incontinence is rare in women suffering from the true urethral syndrome (O'Boyle and Parsons 1979; Jarvis 1982). However, some patients complain of slight urinary loss and Jarvis (1982), studying 33 patients with sensory urgency, observed a positive urilos nappy test in all cases on at least one occasion. He was unable to explain the mechanism of the incontinence in these patients with stable bladders who did not have genuine stress incontinence but suggested that, as the leakage relieved symptoms of suprapubic pain, the incontinence might be a means of reducing discomfort. Bladder retraining may be of considerable benefit in this group of patients (Jarvis 1982; Holmes et al. 1983).

Urethral Hypersensitivity and Bladder Instability

In some patients the urethral syndrome might be expected to occur in conjunction with bladder instability and in these cases it will be difficult, if not impossible, to determine which symptoms relate to which disorder. Urethral sensation associated with bladder instability may indeed be very similar to that experienced in the hypersensitive disorders. Hence some clinicians include such patients under the heading of the urethral syndrome, making a tacit assumption that the two dysfunctional states are linked together. Several experimental studies suggest that this proposition is incorrect.

Sensation from the middle third of the urethra, the apparent site of tenderness as judged by catheterisation (Shah et al. 1983) and area of maximum urethral pressure as measured by profilometry (Raz and Smith 1976), is routed by the pudendal nerve (Nathan 1956; Sundin et al. 1974). Stimulation of this nerve and its branches either by penile squeeze (Kondo et al. 1982) or following anal dilatation (Kock and Pompeius 1963) diminishes rather than enhances detrusor contraction and indeed such a mechanism has been implicated as a cause of urinary retention following anal surgery (Kock and Pompeius 1963). Urethral pressure measurements and electromyographic recordings in patients with bladder instability have shown a *decrease* in pressure and electrical silence to occur before the onset of the detrusor contraction (Low 1977; Webster et al. 1984) and it has been further suggested that urethral *hypo-* rather than *hyper*sensitivity—i.e. poor appreciation of urethral function—may be important in the genesis of some forms of detrusor instability (Hindmarsh et al. 1983; Powell and Feneley 1980). By contrast a significant *delay* in urethral opening prior to micturition is commonly observed in the hypersensitive urethral disorders (O'Boyle and Parsons 1979; see p. 110) and this may in part be related to non-relaxation or spasm of the pelvic floor (Kaplan et al. 1980; Raz and Smith 1976).

In summary, urethral hypersensitivity and bladder instability may co-exist but in many instances are unlikely to bear a cause–effect relationship to one another. Under these complex circumstances rational treatment of a patient with the 'urge syndrome' (sensory or motor) will constitute a major therapeutic challenge to the clinician without access to urodynamic facilities.

Urethral Hypersensitivity and Genuine Stress Incontinence

Urethral hypersensitivity also co-exists with sphincter weakness in some patients with genuine stress incontinence. Although the diagnosis of stress incontinence is easier to make on clinical grounds than other forms of female incontinence (Shepherd et al. 1982) it may still prove difficult to distinguish the symptoms due to the urethral syndrome from symptoms related to sphincter weakness. It is of interest that such patients, if cured of their urethral syndrome, may experience a deterioration in the degree of urinary leakage.

Examination and Routine Investigation

Full clinical examination of the patient with the urethral syndrome will be essentially negative although palpation of the urethra during bimanual examination may reveal mild tenderness of the urethral musculature (Shah et al. 1983). Full blood analysis and tests of renal function will lie within normal limits. Urography, found to be normal in 92% of patients studied by Carson et al. (1980), rarely contributes positively to patient management, although in practice the examination is likely to be requested as part of the general process of diagnosis by exclusion.

Frequency/Volume Chart

Frequency/volume charts are important in the assessment of all females with lower urinary tract symptoms. Typically, the chart in a patient with the urethral syndrome will illustrate frequent voiding during the waking hours whilst nocturia, though present, never attains the relentless pattern observed in interstitial cystitis (Fig. 11.1). Several authors have commented upon the ability of these patients to ignore the call to void if their attention is distracted (Klevmark 1981; O'Boyle and Parsons 1979) and such observations might indicate the relative importance of neurological or psychological factors in the disorder (Klevmark 1981). The charts confirm that patients with the urethral syndrome are rarely incontinent and provide objective proof of symptomatic improvement after therapeutic measures such as urethral dilatation.

Bacteriological Investigation—The Significance of Pyuria

The criteria for excluding bacteriuria as a factor in the aetiology of the urethral syndrome have been defined above and elsewhere in this book (Chaps. 9, 10).

Absence of white cells from the urine of most normal individuals led O'Grady and co-workers (1973) to propose that pyuria is of some significance even when appropriate tests have failed to identify a cause for the condition. In support of this contention it was observed that if cultures were performed over an extended period 'abacteriuric' patients with pyuria were on occasion found to excrete bacteria; that is, the patients when originally seen were 'between infections.' Hence some cases of sterile pyuria could be reclassified as cases of bacterial cystitis.

Specialised culture techniques may be required to explain the presence of pyuria in other circumstances. A study in patients with sterile bladder urine revealed *Chlamydia trachomatis* in 10 of 16 patients with pyuria but in only one of 16 patients without white cells in the urine (Stamm et al. 1980). Fastidious carbon dioxide-dependent organisms, chiefly lactobacilli, have been suggested as a cause of the urethral syndrome by Maskell et al. (1979), who further noted that only 66% of infected patients had pyuria. Other workers, however, found no significant difference between the isolation rate of lactobacilli and other organisms in urine cultures from healthy women and from women with frequency and dysuria (Brumfitt et al. 1981).

In summary, although thorough investigation of abacteriuric patients with pyuria will identify a cause for the leucocyte response in a number of cases there will remain some pyuric patients in whom the cause of the urethral syndrome cannot presently be identified.

Bacteriological Investigation—The Significance of Introital Colonisation

The role of introital infection in the genesis of the urethral syndrome remains unclear. A concept of colonisation, transfer (faecal organism to introitus, introitus to urethra, urethra to bladder) and impaired elimination was advanced by O'Grady to explain the occurrence of urethral symptoms in some women whose midstream (VB2) urine remained sterile. It was postulated that symptomatic patients whose urethras become colonised but in whom upward migration of organisms into the bladder was prevented by defence mechanisms might be recognised as suffering from the urethral syndrome (O'Grady et al. 1970). However, introital or urethral colonisation with *E. coli* does not necessarily lead to urinary tract symptomatology and it has been observed that significant numbers (43%) of patients with recurrent infections do not have such introital isolates (Stamey and Sexton 1975). Furthermore, introital coliforms are found in 23% of asymptomatic control women (O'Grady et al. 1970).

The relationship of introital colonisation to inflammatory urethral change was further studied by Charlton et al. (1973). Enterobacteria were isolated from 25 of 40 patients with the urethral syndrome; 16 of these 25 were symptomatic at the time of the examination, but in only 6 could concurrent inflammatory change be identified in the urethral mucosa.

IF YOU ARE TO ATTEND FOR AN I.V.P. – THAT IS AN X–RAY OF YOUR KIDNEYS AND BLADDER – DO NOT KEEP ANY RECORD ON THE DATE THAT YOU ATTEND FOR THE X–RAY EXAMINATION.

	DAY	TIME / VOLUME DAY TIME (measure volumes in mls, ccs or fl. oz.)	TIME / VOLUME NIGHT TIME	
1500	1	7am/7 8·45/5 10/4 11·35/5 12·25/7 2/3 5·15pm/7 7pm/3 9·15pm/5 10·30/4	5·15am/9	10/1
2500	2	6am/5 6·25/4 6·55/3 8am/5 8·45/10 9·20/8 10·15/10 11·20/9 12md/4 2·30/5 4pm/7 5·30/5 9pm/5 10·30/5	4·30am/8	14/1
2250	3	6·15/5 7/5 8am/5 9·10am/10 9·55/10 10·20/5 10·55/7 11·25/5 12·45/4 2·45/4 4pm/5 6·30/3 9pm/5 11·30/4		14/0
1220	4	6·30am/8 7/5 8am/3 9·30/5 11·15/3 12·30/4 4pm/4 5·30/4 8·30/5 10·30pm/3		10/0
1860	5	6am/10 6·30/5 6·55/3 8·30/10 9·45/9 10·35/4 10·55/3 12/9 12·50pm/3 3·10/5 5·30/3 7pm/3 9·30/3 11/3		14/0
2700	6	6·50am/7 7·05/16 8am/5 8·50/8 9am/7 10am/5 10·30/3 12·50pm/10 3·20/9 4·15/4 5·30/3 7·30/6 10·15/10 11·15/5	5·45/6	14/1
1600	7	7·15/16 7·35/3 8·25/5 9·45/6 11·05am/5 12·55pm/6 1·35/7 2·30/3 4·30/5 6·45/3 8pm/3 11pm/8 11·30/3		13/0

a

Fig. 11.1 **a** Frequency volume chart in a 35-year-old woman with the apyuric urethral syndrome. Intense daytime frequency and little nocturia illustrate the 'psychosomatic' form of micturition habit. As in many cases this patient was drinking moderate amounts of fluids in an attempt to diminish the urethral 'niggle'. (Volumes recorded in fluid ounces; 1 fl. oz. = 30 ml.). **b** Chart from 31-year-old with pyuric urethral syndrome. Antibiotics were commenced on day 2, leading to considerable improvement in frequency and volume voided.

IF YOU ARE TO ATTEND FOR AN I.V.P. – THAT IS AN X–RAY OF YOUR KIDNEYS AND BLADDER – DO NOT KEEP ANY RECORD ON THE DATE THAT YOU ATTEND FOR THE X–RAY EXAMINATION.

DAY	TIME / VOLUME DAY TIME (measure volumes in mls, ccs or fl. oz.)	TIME / VOLUME NIGHT TIME
1	7.30 am/140 9am/160 9.30/240 10.20/175 11.05/70 12.17/70 1.35/40 2.40/100 4pm/150 6pm – 170 9pm 100 11pm 100	
2	7.15/350 9am/150 10.00/100 2pm/140 4pm/180 5.30/250 10.20/325	
3	7.30/350 9.00/250 12/* 3pm/200 10.30/300	
4	7.30/325 11.20/200 4.30/180 9pm/350	
5	7.30/350 12.30pm/250 5.30/300 8pm/300 10.30/230	
6	7.30/400 1pm/250 8.30/230 11pm/300	
7	7.30/300 10.30/200 12.00/150 2pm/150 7pm/150 9pm/100.	

Fig. 11.1b

It may be concluded that while the concept of restricted colonisation and transfer postulated by O'Grady may be a cause of urinary tract infection in some patients and the urethral syndrome in others, there remain a number of inconsistencies in the theory for which there are as yet no explanations. A positive introital culture may be obtained in normal asymptomatic women and such a finding therefore will not exclude the diagnosis of the urethral syndrome in a patient whose fractional urines confirm abacteruria.

Psychological Investigation

Several workers have investigated the possible role of psychological factors in the aetiology (Carson et al. 1980) and clinical expression (Kaplan et al. 1980) of the urethral syndrome. Psychological history taking is naturally time consuming and best carried out at a specific patient interview when specialised questionnaires can be filled in at the patient's leisure.

Using the Minnesota Multi-Phasic Personality Inventory (MMPI) 56 patients with the urethral syndrome scored significantly higher on scales of hypochondriasis, hysteria and schizophrenia than did control patients (Carson et al. 1980). These authors concluded that in this group of patients reassurance, in combination with psychiatric consultation when necessary, was as likely to prove beneficial as other more conventional forms of therapy such as urethral dilatation. However, the further suggestion of these authors and others (Zufall 1963) that certain invasive diagnostic measures could be omitted in these patients cannot be supported.

Urethral Sensitivity Tests

The highly subjective nature of the patients' symptoms have been responsible in the past for much of the diagnostic confusion that surrounds the sensory disorders. The advent of sophisticated electronic techniques for both pressure measurement and electrostimulation have allowed an opportunity for objective measurement of physiological change in these conditions, although it will be recognised that the tests continue to rely on the patient's subjective perception of her condition during the procedure.

A series of young female patients aged 18–33 years complaining of frequency, dysuria and suprapubic discomfort were investigated by Powell et al. (1981) to assess the role of urethral hypersensitivity in the genesis of the urethral syndrome. Cystometric investigation revealed reduced bladder capacity (range 80–375 ml, mean 227 ml) but no evidence of instability. Urine flow rates were diminished with an interrupted pattern of voiding leading to marked hesitancy and prolongation of micturition in many cases (see also p. 107).

Urethral sensitivity recordings were undertaken in these patients according to the method described by Powell and Feneley (1980). The results demonstrated that the patients had significantly reduced urethral sensitivity thresholds, i.e. urethral hypersensitivity, when they were compared with similar groups of patients with either genuine stress incontinence or detrusor instability (Table 11.1). Similar findings were first described by Keisswetter (1977), who showed

Table 11.1. Urethral sensitivity in females with stress incontinence, bladder instability or urethral syndrome, and in a control group

Condition	n	Electrosensitivity (mA)	±1SD
Normal	6	4.9	0.9
Stress incontinence	5	5.6	1.1
Bladder instability	8	6.4	1.9
Urethral syndrome	10	2.0	1.7

that the urgency syndrome in the adult female was characterised by a low perception threshold in the posterior urethra whilst the bladder electrosensitivity threshold was within the normal range. In particular, 39 out of 40 patients with sensory urgency were shown to have urethral hypersensitivity. More recently Opsomer et al. (1983), while confirming these findings, also demonstrated that bladder electrosensitivity thresholds were reduced in some patients who had sensory urgency and urethral hypersensitivity.

Endoscopic Observations

Cysto-urethroscopy is essential before the diagnosis of the urethral syndrome can be established. The examination should be performed under general anaesthetic so as to exclude all forms of inflammatory or neoplastic disease. The reduced functional capacity of fibrotic bladder conditions such as radiation bladder disease or 'classical' interstitial cystitis may be distinguished from the normal capacity of the anaesthetised patient with the urethral syndrome (Klevmark 1981; Powell and Yeates 1982).

The female urethra is often difficult to visualise through a standard endoscope and a special urethral instrument is required for adequate inspection. The mucosa of both urethra and bladder should be essentially normal although non-specific oedematous changes are occasionally seen in the folds of the urethra. The significance of occasional haemorrhagic areas seen on the wall of the normal capacity bladder remains unknown.

The Urge Syndrome

This non-specific term has been used to describe patients with a multitude of abnormalities of the lower urinary tract, including the poorly compliant bladder, the unstable bladder, the hypersensitive bladder and the incompetent bladder neck. Urodynamic studies are essential to distinguish between these groups of patients, all of whom may describe symptoms of urgency referrable to the urethral zone (Holmes et al. 1983).

Bladder retraining (Frewin 1980) has been shown to be successful in treating patients with sensory urgency. Results both in the short term (Jarvis 1982) and after longer periods (Holmes et al. 1983) demonstrate the importance of making a clear distinction between these patients and those with motor urgency (bladder instability). In the latter group treatment by retraining is unlikely to be successful in more than half the cases (Holmes et al. 1983).

Powell and Yeates (1982) have adopted a plan to discriminate between the various causes of frequency and dysuria in female patients with the 'urge syndrome' (Fig. 11.2). Following the exclusion of organic disease, bladder capacity is measured at physiological pressures (10 cm of water) under general anaesthetic. Patients with reduced capacity are considered to have an interstitial cystitis or allied condition; those with normal capacity are subjected to urodynamic investigation. Inflow studies in these cases will reveal either phasic bladder instability or stable filling characteristics. The latter group is subdivided according to whether the attention of the patient can be distracted during filling or whether urethral hypersensitivity precludes the attainment of a normal bladder capacity. It is acknowledged that the latter two groups represent in all probability opposite ends of the same spectrum within which clear distinctions are not always possible (Powell and Yeates 1982; Holmes et al. 1983). Bladder retraining should succeed in both groups (Jarvis 1982) but, as might be expected, is most successful in those patients in whom the aetiology of the disorder is likely to be of psychological origin.

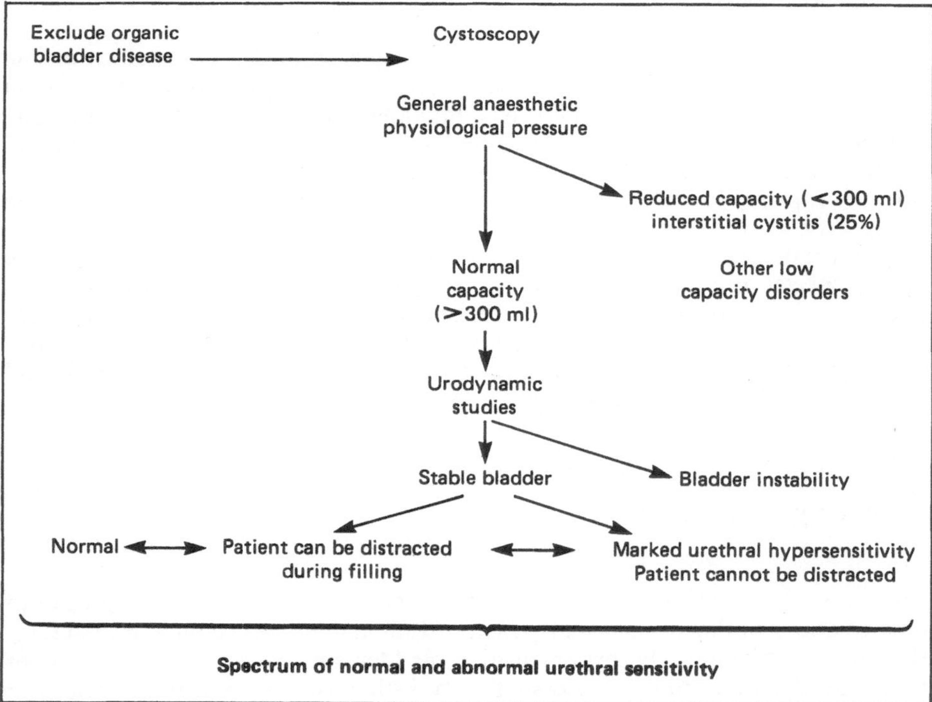

Fig. 11.2. The 'urge syndrome'. The rational plan devised by Powell and Yeates (1982) excludes first those with reduced capacity under anaesthetic and then patients with bladder instability. The remaining patients constitute part of a spectrum which ranges from the normal to intense urethral hypersensitivity where the attention of the patient cannot be distracted during filling studies.

References

BMJ (1977) The urethral syndrome. Br Med J II:593–594

Brumfitt W, Hamilton-Miller JMT, Ludlam H, Gooding A, (1981) Lactobacilli do not cause frequency and dysuria syndrome. Lancet II:393–395

Carson CC, Segura JW, Osborne DM (1980) Evaluation and treatment of the female urethral syndrome. J Urol 124: 609–610

Charlton CAC, Cattell WR, Canti G, Grottick J, O'Grady FW (1973) The non urethral syndrome. In: Brumfitt W, Asscher AW (eds) Urinary tract infection. Oxford University Press, Oxford, pp 173–177

Frewin WK (1980) The management of urgency and frequency of micturition. Br J Urol 52:367–369

Hindmarsh JR, Gosling PT, Deane AM (1983) Bladder instability. Is the primary defect in the urethra? Br J Urol 55:648–651

Holmes DM, Stone AR, Bary PR, Richards CJ, Stephenson TP (1983) Bladder training—3 years on. Br J Urol 55: 660–664

Jarvis GJ (1982) The management of urinary incontinence due to primary vesical sensory urgency by bladder drill. Br J Urol 54: 374–376

Kaplan WE, Firlit CF, Schoenberg HW (1980) The female urethral syndrome: External sphincter spasm as etiology. J Urol 124:48–49

Kiesswetter H (1977) Mucosal sensory threshold of the urinary bladder and urethra measured electrically. Urol Int 32:437–448

Klevmark B (1981) Hyperactive neurogenic bladder studied with physiological filling rates. Scand J Urol Nephrol (Suppl) 60:55–56

Kock NG, Pompeius R (1963) Inhibition of vesical motor activity induced by anal stimulation. Acta Chir Scand 126:244–250

Kondo A, Otari T, Takita T (1982) Suppression of bladder instability by penile squeeze. Br J Urol 54:360–362

Low JA (1977) Urethral behaviour during the involuntary detrusor contraction. Am J Obstet Gynecol 128:32–42

Mabry EW, Carson CC, Older RA (1981) Evaluation of women with chronic voiding discomfort. Urology 18: 244–246

Maskell R, Pead L, Allen J (1979) The puzzle of "urethral syndrome": a possible answer? Lancet I: 1058–1059

Meadow SR, White RHR, Johnston NM (1969) Prevalence of symptomless urinary tract disease in Birmingham school children. I—Pyuria and bacteruria. Br Med J 3:81–84

Nathan PW (1956) Sensations associated with micturition. Br J Urol 28:126–131

O'Boyle PJ, Parsons KF (1979) Primary vesical sensory urgency. A clinical trial of bromocriptine. Br J Urol 51: 200–203

O'Grady FW, Richards B, McSherry MA, O'Farrell SM, Cattell WR (1970) Introital enterobateria, urinary infection and the urethral syndrome. Lancet II:1208–1210

O'Grady FW, Charlton CAC, Fry IK, McSherry A, Cattell WR (1973) Natural history of intractable 'cystitis' in women referred to a special clinic. In: Brumfitt W, Asscher AW (eds) Urinary tract infection. Oxford University Press, Oxford, pp 81–91

Opsomer RJ, Gerstenberg TC, Klarskov P, Hald T (1983) The electric sensibility threshold in the bladder and the urethra. Paper presented at the XIIIth Meeting of the International Continence Society

Powell PH, Feneley RCL (1980) The role of urethral sensation in clinical urology. Br J Urol 52:539–541

Powell PH, George NJR, Smith PJB, Feneley RCL (1981) The hypersensitive female urethra—a cause of recurrent frequency and dysuria. In: Proceedings of the XIth Meeting of the International Continence Society, pp 81–82

Powell PH, Yeates WK (1982) The clinical value of bladder capacity measurement at physiological pressure under anaesthesia. Br J Urol 54:650–652

Raz S, Smith RB (1976) External sphincter spasticity syndrome in female patients. J Urol 115:443–446

Shah PJR, Whiteside CGC, Turner-Warwick RT, Milroy EJG (1983) The hypersensitive female urethra—A catheter diagnosis? In: Proceedings of the XIIIth Meeting of the International Continence Society, pp 202–204

Shepherd AM, Powell PH, Ball AJ (1982) The place of urodynamic studies in the investigation and treatment of female urinary tract symptoms. J Obstet Gynaecol 3:123–125
Smith PJB (1979) The management of the urethral syndrome. Br J Hosp Med 22:578–587
Smith PJB, Powell PH, George NJR, Kirk D (1981) Urethrolysis in the management of females with recurrent frequency and dysuria. Br J Urol 53:634–636
Stamey TA, Sexton CC (1975) The role of vaginal colonization with enterobacteriaceae in recurrent urinary infections. J Urol 113:214–217
Stamm WE, Wagner KF, Ansel R, Alexander ER, Turck M, Counts GW, Holmes KK (1980) Causes of the acute urethral syndrome in women. N Engl J Med 303:409–415
Sundin T, Carlsson GA, Kock NG (1974) Detrusor inhibition induced from mechanical stimulation of the anal region and from electrical stimulation of pudendal nerve afferents. Invest Urol 11:374–378
Webster JR (1975) Combined video/pressure/flow cystourethrography in female patients with voiding disturbances. Urology 5:209–215
Webster GD, Sihelnik SA, Stone AR (1984) Female urinary incontinence: Incidence, identification and characteristics of detrusor instability. Neurourol Urodyn 3:235–242
Zufall R (1963) Treatment of the urethral syndrome in women. JAMA 184:894–896

Chapter 12

Structure of the Trigone and Urethra in the Urethral Syndrome

J.S. Dixon

Pseudo-membranous Trigonitis

Pseudo-membranous trigonitis is a change which may be observed in the mucosa overlying the trigone in patients with the urethral syndrome (Henry and Fox 1971) but is also seen within the bladder of normal asymptomatic women (i.e. women cystoscoped for reasons unrelated to the lower urinary tract). The relationship of this anatomical variant to symptom complexes arising from the lower urinary tract thus remains a matter for debate (Davies and Hunt 1981).

The characteristic cystoscopic lesion of pseudo-membranous trigonitis is restricted to the trigone of the bladder and consists of greyish white patches which are sometimes surrounded with a hyperaemic cuff (Henry and Fox 1971). The patches present a characteristic cobblestone or pallisade appearance when viewed obliquely through an endoscope (Fig. 12.1) and commonly extend as a sheet from the proximal urethra onto the trigone but may then break up into discrete metaplastic islands surrounded by normal trigonal epithelium (Tyler 1962). The condition was first described by Heymann (1905) as 'trigonal cystitis'

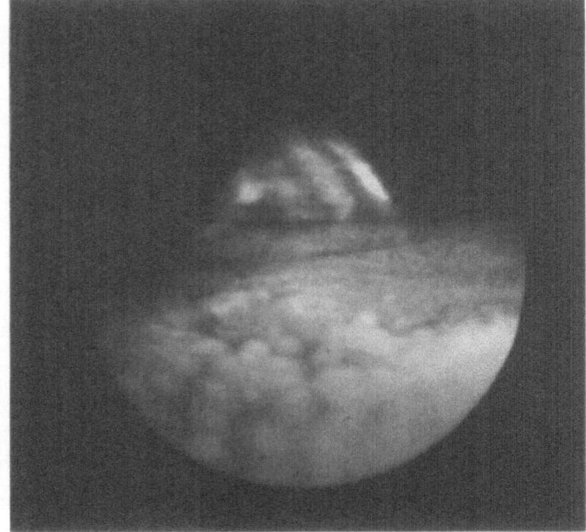

Fig. 12.1. Characteristic appearance of pseudo-membranous trigonitis seen through 30° endoscope. The 'cobblestone' change in the mucosa can be seen extending to the edge of the trigone. Reflected light from the biopsy forceps is seen superiorly.

and has since been given various names including pseudo-membranous trigonitis (Ryall 1929), urethrotrigonitis (Clark and Gherardi 1962) and vaginal or squamous metaplasia of the trigonal epithelium (Cifuentes 1947; Ney and Ehrlich 1955).

Histological examination of the trigonal epithelium from such patients demonstrates a non-keratinising squamous metaplasia, the epithelium being thicker than the normal transitional type (Fig. 12.2). The cells are frequently vacuolated and contain quantities of glycogen, having an appearance similar to vaginal epithelium (Fig. 12.3). The edge of the lesion shows a sudden transition from vaginal epithelium to the transitional form. The lamina propria frequently shows marked venous dilatation but there is usually no significant inflammatory cell infiltration.

A recent study using scanning electron microscopy shows that the superficial cells of the thickened squamous epithelium of the trigone have either a microridged, microvillus or mixed pattern. Some cells have a cobblestone appearance with long clubbed microvilli and resemble the cells observed in malignant and pre-malignant states (Davies and Hunt 1981). Such observations presumably reflect the non-specific nature of these changes, as malignancy is considered not to develop in pseudo-membranous trigonitis (Weiner et al. 1979).

Pseudo-membranous trigonitis is found almost exclusively in female patients (Ney and Ehrlich 1955) and may result from oestrogenic stimulation upon the epithelium of the trigone. The condition is rarely, if ever, seen before the

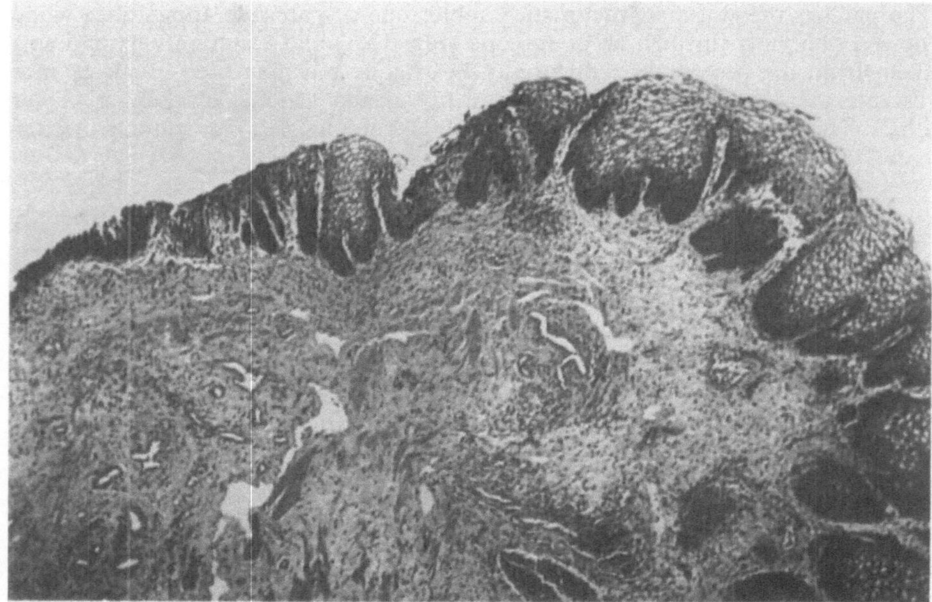

Fig. 12.2. Biopsy from the trigone showing squamous metaplasia and junction with normal urothelium towards the left of the field. Haematoxylin and eosin, ×200

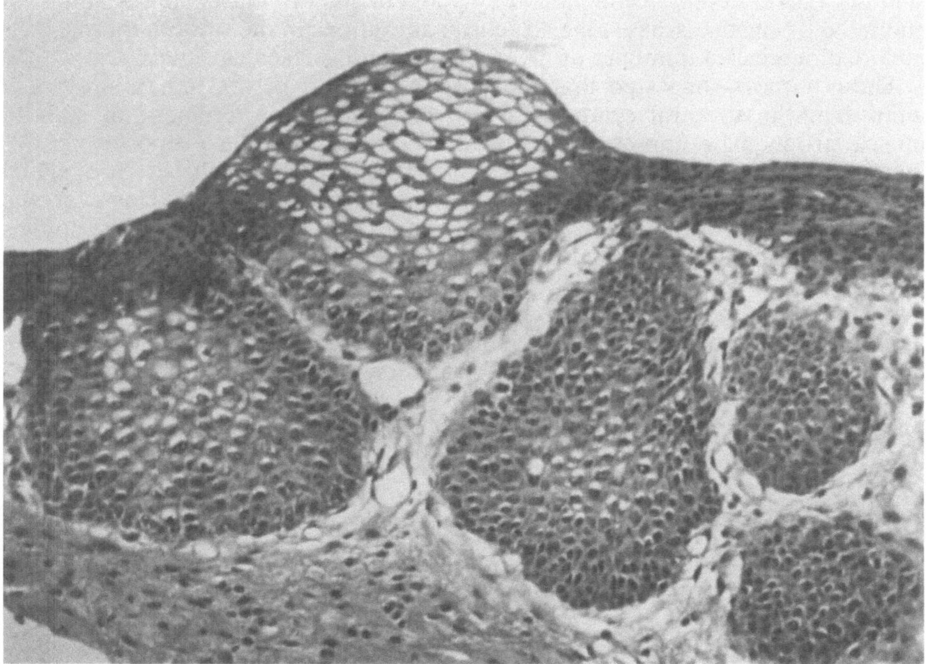

Fig. 12.3. Squamous metaplasia of trigone at high magnification. Note the large perinuclear clear areas giving the appearance of a 'vaginal' type of epithelium. Haematoxylin and eosin, ×400

menarche and becomes less common after the menopause (Cifuentes 1947; Ney and Ehrlich 1955; Clark and Cherardi 1962).

Further evidence of the oestrogenic influence on the trigonal epithelium was provided by Ney and Ehrlich (1955), who observed growth in the size of the pseudo-membranous patches in patients on oestrogen therapy, and Tyler (1962), who observed similar changes in the trigone of a man on stilboestrol for carcinoma of the prostate.

Urethral Morphology

The suggestion that the urethra may represent an obstructive barrier to micturition has led some authorities to remove urethral tissue in an attempt to cure the patient's symptom complex (Richardson 1969). These operations provide an opportunity to examine carefully the morphology of the urethral wall in the patient with urethral hypersensitivity.

Tissue removed from 50 patients with the urethral syndrome during Richardson urethroplasty was examined by light and electron microscopy (Splatt and Weedon 1981). A significant increase in fibrous tissue in the urethrovaginal septum was observed, accompanied by a loss of smooth muscle fibres and focal clumping of elastic tissues. Fine structural alterations in the smooth muscle cells included decreased numbers of myofilaments and surface caveolae.

These authors suggested that the normal anatomy of the female urethra is altered in the urethral syndrome, with collagenous replacement of smooth muscle producing a non-compliant urethra. Evans (1971) also reported on this increase in collagen by measuring hydroxyprolene values in the urethrovaginal septum of patients with the urethral syndrome coming to autopsy. However, the cause and extent of the urethral fibrosis remain open to question as the studies were not well controlled and most concerned a comparison between middle aged women (40–50 years) and cadaver material of unspecified origin (Splatt and Weedon 1977, 1981). It remains possible that there may be an increase in fibrous tissue in these patients but equal weight must be given to the theories invoking muscle spasm as the cause (or effect) of the syndrome (Raz and Smith 1976; Kaplan et al. 1980) particularly since psychological (Carson et al. 1980) and diazepam therapy (Kaplan et al. 1980) appear to produce relief in many patients.

References

Carson CC, Segura JW, Osborne DM (1980) Evaluation and treatment of the female urethral syndrome. J Urol 124:609–610

Cifuentes L (1947) Epithelium of vaginal type in the female trigone: The clinical problem of trigonitis. J Urol 57: 1028–1037

Clarke BG, Cherardi GJ (1962) Urethrotrigonitis or epidermidization of the trigone of the bladder: A histologic, bacteriologic and clinical study. J Urol 87:545–548

Davies R, Hunt AC (1981) Surface topography of the female bladder trigone. J Clin Pathol 34:308–313

Evans AT (1971) Aetiology of urethral syndrome: Preliminary report. J Urol 105:245–250

Henry L, Fox M (1971) Histological findings in pseudo-membranous trigonitis. J Clin Pathol 24:605–608

Heymann A (1905) Die Cystitis Trigoni der Frau. Zentralbl Kr Harn Sex Org 16:422–433

Kaplan WE, Firlit CF, Schoenberg HW (1980) The female urethral syndrome: External sphincter spasm as etiology. J Urol 124:48–49

Ney C, Ehrlich JC (1955) Squamous epithelium in the trigone of the human female urinary bladder. J Urol 73:809–819

Raz S, Smith RB (1976) External sphincter spasticity syndrome in female patients. J Urol 115:443–446

Richardson FH (1969) External urethroplasty in women: Technique and clinic evaluation. J Urol 101:709–723

Ryall EC (1929) Pseudo-membranous trigonitis. Br J Urol 1:255–257

Splatt AJ, Weedon D (1977) The urethral syndrome: Experience with the Richardson urethroplasty. Br J Urol 49:173–176

Splatt AJ, Weedon D (1981) The urethral syndrome: Morphological studies. Br J Urol 53:263–265

Tyler DE (1962) Stratified squamous epithelium in the vesical trigone and urethra: Findings correlated with the menstrual cycle and age. Am J Anat 111:319–325

Weiner DP, Koss LG, Sablay B, Freed SZ (1979) The prevalence and significance of Brunn's nests, cystitis cystica and squamous metaplasia in normal bladders. J Urol 122:317–321

Chapter 13

Urethral Syndrome—Urodynamic Studies

N.J.R. George

Introduction

A diagnosis of the urethral syndrome requires prior urodynamic investigation as bladder stability cannot be accurately predicted by symptoms alone (Shepherd et al. 1982). In a number of patients bladder instability or genuine stress incontinence may occur in association with the urethral syndrome and the urodynamic picture in such cases is likely to be complex, see p. 93. In an effort to identify the urodynamic pattern that characterises the uncomplicated syndrome this account deals with a study on 16 younger women in whom other abnormalities of the lower urinary tract were absent. The mean age of the patients was 26 years but nevertheless in most cases symptoms had been present for a number of years prior to investigation.

Urodynamic Observations

Studies consisted of free flow rate, measurement of urethral pressure profile, bladder filling and voiding cystometry. All tests were performed by the same investigator under identical conditions in a warm, quiet environment.

Free Flow Rate

Considerable variation in the maxium free flow rates occurred although in the majority of patients the values were reduced when compared with the flow rate in control women of the same age (mean 16 ml/s, range 5–35). Parodoxically some patients, presumably over-anxious to comply with pre-test instructions, suppressed their desire to void and over-filled their bladder. In these cases the flow rate was often prolonged and interrupted (Fig. 13.1). The ability of these patients to 'hold on' despite persistent urethral sensation was noted by O'Boyle and Parsons (1979).

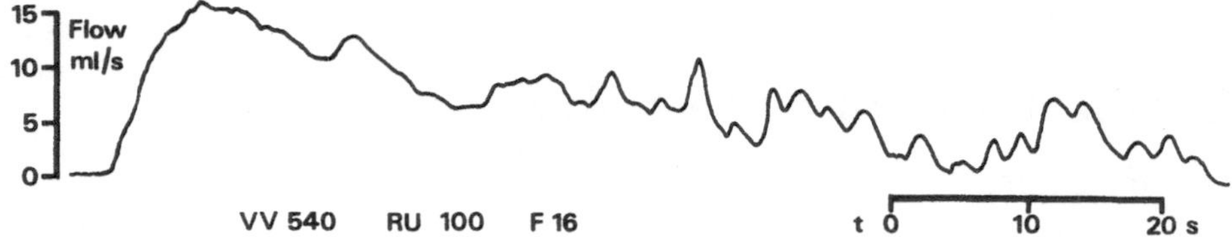

Fig. 13.1. Apyuric urethral syndrome. The patient, aged 28, arrived overfull at the Urodynamic Unit and flow was prolonged (1 min 20 s) and moderately painful. Residual urine was not present at other times when tested by catheterisation.

Urethral Pressure Profile

Catheterization of the patient with the urethral syndrome must be undertaken with extreme care as the urethra is frequently tender to touch and acute discomfort will of necessity preclude further urodynamic investigation. Some authors consider the painful urethra to be a sign of diagnostic importance in the urethral syndrome (Shah et al. 1983). The urethral pressure profile presents typical characteristics (Fig. 13.2) and the mean maximum urethral closure pressure in the patients studied was 103 cm of water, range 68–128, a level in excess of the normal age-matched mean (88 cm of water, Abrams et al. 1983). Most workers agree that these observations result from spasm of periurethral striated (pelvic floor) muscle (Kaplan et al. 1980; Carson et al. 1980; Raz and Smith 1976). Few patients are able to increase significantly the maximum profile pressure during voluntary squeeze (Fig. 13.2).

Inflow Cystometrogram

During filling the cystometrogram is, by definition, stable in the urethral syndrome and the patient experiences an early first desire to void. In the study referred to above the first desire to micturate was noted in the majority of patients between 80 and 100 ml and the mean capacity at the normal desire to void was 227 ml. Despite the intense periurethral desire experienced by some patients pressure rise during filling did not exceed 10 cm of water ('superstable'),

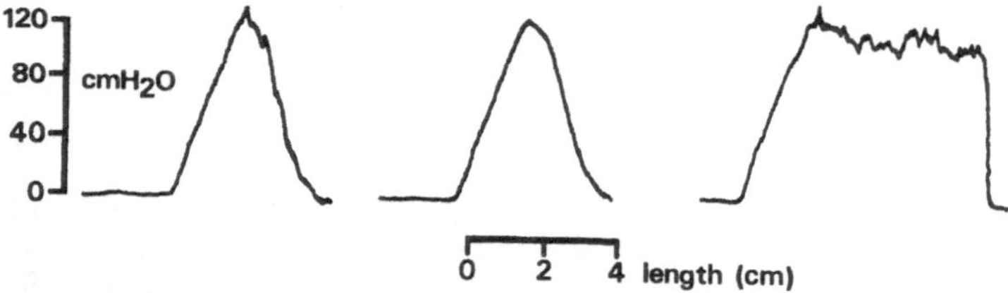

Fig. 13.2. Urethral pressure profile in urethral syndrome. Nulliparous patient aged 21 with 3 years' history of frequency. Urethra tender to catheterisation. *Left* two resting profiles and *right* squeeze profile. Voluntary contraction is unlikely to be the cause of the raised pressure noted in the resting profiles as the shape is reproducible over extended periods of time. Maximum voluntary contraction of the pelvic floor cannot be maintained over such periods and the shape of the profile might be expected to be irregular, as seen *right*.

a finding in agreement with that of O'Boyle and Parsons (1979). If the patient's attention can be distracted during the test it may be possible to fill the bladder to a normal volume and this observation has been used to distinguish between the different forms of sensory disorders (Klevmark 1981).

Micturating Cystometrogram

Satisfactory studies of micturition in patients with the urethral syndrome can only be obtained if the patient voids alone in a quiet room. In the present series of patients mean intrinsic detrusor pressure and maximum flow rate were 30 cm of water and 13 ml/s respectively (Figs. 13.3, 13.4).

The urine flow rate, considerably reduced when compared with that observed in normal women of the same age, is responsible for the widely held belief that these patients have a degree of outflow tract obstruction (Richardson 1969; Splatt and Weedon 1977). Pressure–flow studies demonstrate conclusively that this low flow results from a normal or, more usually, an under-active detrusor

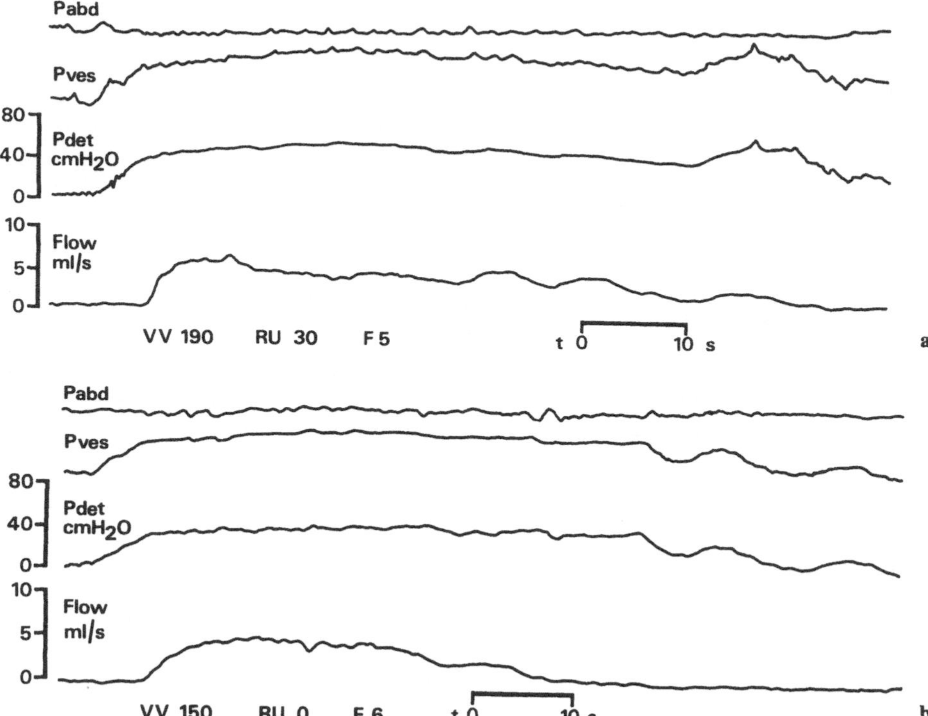

Fig. 13.3. **a** Micturating cystometrogram, female aged 24. Poor flow associated with a weak detrusor contraction. Micturition takes one minute. **b** Three months after urethral dilatation total flow rate is little improved but voiding is completed in a shorter time according to the patient's subjective account. Objective evidence for this improvement is lacking due to different voided volumes. *Pabd*, intra-abdominal pressure; *Pves*, intravesical pressure; *Pdet*, subtracted detrusor pressure.

contraction and is not associated with raised pressure as would be expected in true obstruction. These observations are in agreement with those of Rees et al. (1976), who were unable to demonstrate obstruction in 200 patients with frequency and dysuria. O'Boyle and Parsons (1979) similarly noted voiding pressures to be normal in a study of 21 patients with sensory urgency.

The effect of urethral dilatation in two patients with the urethral syndrome is illustrated in Figs. 13.3 and 13.4. In one case the results were objectively disappointing although subjectively the patient reported that voiding had improved by virtue of the reduced time that was required to pass urine. This type of response is common although occasionally an objective increase in flow rate is obtained (Fig. 13.4).

The factors responsible for the urodynamic findings in patients with the urethral syndrome remain obscure but it is possible that the hypersensitive urethra in some way predisposes both to excessive pelvic floor tension and the 'poorly relaxed' pattern of micturition observed in the majority of cases. Urethral discomfort during voiding is not, however, a particular cause for

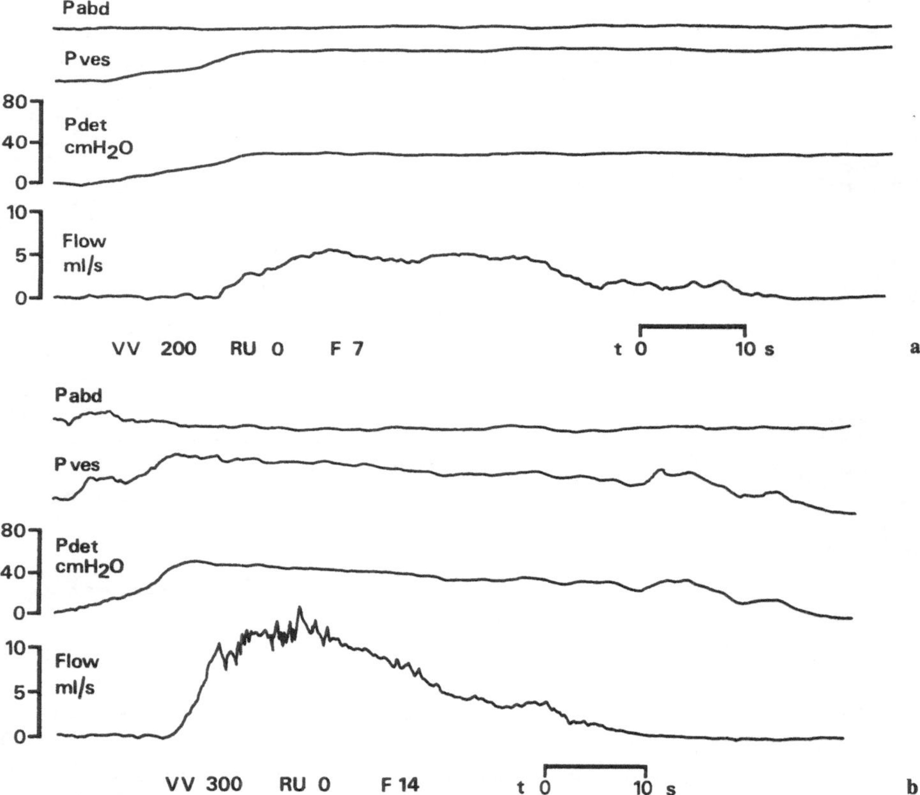

Fig. 13.4. **a** Low pressure, low flow trace in woman of 44. Micturition lasting 50 s. **b** Two weeks after dilatation flow rate showed considerable improvement. It is notable that subtracted voiding pressure has also risen, possibly implying a more effective detrusor contraction. *Pabd*, intra-abdominal pressure; *Pves*, intravesical pressure; *Pdet*, subtracted detrusor pressure.

complaint in many patients with the syndrome and thus pain cannot always be implicated as a cause of the condition (Kaplan et al. 1980; Raz and Smith 1976). Nevertheless, it would seem reasonable to suppose that if hypertonicity of the pelvic floor during voiding is of importance such inappropriate neurological activity might also explain the inability to maintain an adequate detrusor contraction. Organic neurological disease is, however, very unlikely to be present in the urethral syndrome as the condition responds to central and local relaxant agents such as diazepam (Raz and Smith 1976) or to psychological modes of therapy (Carson et al. 1980). A very similar effect may be observed in male patients with prostatodynia or the anxious bladder syndrome.

References

Abrams PH, Feneley RCL, Torrens M (1983) Urodynamics. Springer, Berlin Heidelberg New York, pp 48–61

Carson CC, Segura JW, Osborne DM (1980) Evaluation and treatment of the female urethral syndrome. J Urol 124:609–610

Kaplan WE, Firlit CF, Schoenberg HW (1980) The female urethral syndrome: External sphincter spasm as etiology. J Urol 124:48–49

Klevmark B (1981) Hyperactive neurogenic bladder studied with physiological filling rates. Scand J Urol Nephrol (Suppl) 60:55–56

O'Boyle PJ, Parsons KF (1979) Primary vesical sensory urgency. A clinical trial of bromocriptine. Br J Urol 51:200–203

Raz S, Smith RB (1976) External sphincter spasticity syndrome in female patients. J Urol 115:443–446

Rees DLP, Whitfield HN, Islam AKMS, Doyle PT, Mayo ME, Wickham JEA (1976) Urodynamic findings in adult females with frequency and dysuria. Br J Urol 47:853–860

Richardson FH (1969) External urethroplasty in women: Technique and clinic evaluation. J Urol 101:709–723

Shah PJR, Whiteside CGC, Turner-Warwick RT, Milroy EJG (1983) The hypersensitive female urethra—A catheter diagnosis? Paper presented at the XIIIth meeting of the International Continence Society

Shepherd AM, Powell PH, Ball AJ (1982) The place of urodynamic studies in the investigation and treatment of female urinary tract symptoms. J Obstet Gynaecol 3:123–125

Splatt AJ, Weedon D (1977) The urethral syndrome: Experience with the Richardson urethroplasty. Br J Urol 49:173–176

Chapter 14

Treatment of the Urethral Syndrome

M. Tasker

Introduction

The patients to be considered for treatment in this section fall conveniently into pyuric (persistent or intermittent) and apyuric groups according to the definition of the urethral syndrome described above (p. 91). Those patients in whom significant pyuria occurs will be the subject of intensive microbiological investigation in an attempt to isolate the suspected organism and it is recognised that longitudinal studies will be required to obtain positive results in the 'between infections' patients (O'Grady et al. 1973). Additionally, *Chlamydia trachomatis* will be isolated from a number of cases (Stamm et al. 1980) but there will remain a significant minority whose urethral syndrome is associated with a pyuria for which no cause can be found. Patients whose urine never contains white cells constitute the 'hard core' of the urethral syndrome and it would appear that infection is unlikely to be implicated as the factor responsible for the symptom complex in these cases (O'Grady et al. 1973).

The division into pyuric and apyuric groups thus forms a natural basis upon which to plan therapeutic schedules though most clinicians openly admit that in many cases the difficulty in obtaining satisfactory symptomatic resolution often leads to illogical modes of treatment. Furthermore, it must be borne in mind that the natural history of both forms of the condition is one of exacerbation and remission, thus making the benefits of treatment difficult to evaluate and confirming the need for controlled clinical trials of therapy. Discrepancies in the definition of urethral syndrome add further to the difficulties of the clinician attempting to assess the efficacy of treatment regimes reported in the literature.

The possible forms of treatment for the urethral syndrome are:

1. General measures
2. Antibiotics
3. Pharmacological and surgical treatment for the urethral syndrome
4. Other surgical techniques
5. Psychological aspects and bladder training

In general, patients with pyuria might be expected to respond to the first two measures whilst patients with acellular urine would require alternative forms of treatment (Stamm et al. 1980, 1981). However, as noted above, theory and practice do not always go hand in hand in dealing with the urethral syndrome and most patients will undertake a variety of therapeutic regimes before a satisfactory solution to the problem is found.

General Measures

Many women become embarrassed and demoralised by the symptoms of the urethral syndrome. It is important to stress the benign nature of the condition and that progression to serious renal disease will not occur. A simple explanation of the symptoms should be given in order to aid the patient's understanding of her own condition. A high daily fluid intake (2–3 litres) is recommended. This dilutes the bladder urine and promotes a wash-out of urethral organisms (Asscher 1978) which, though excluded by definition from VB1 urine, nevertheless may lead to urethral symptoms by virtue of intermittent urethral colonisation. Hydration therapy also demands that the patient makes an effort to retain greater volumes of urine within the bladder in order to prevent intolerable frequency and this is in itself a form of bladder retraining. Excess tea, coffee or alcohol may act as an irritant to the urethra and should be restricted. Introital hygiene is important, and a few women improve when they stop using vaginal deodorants, bubble baths and biological washing powders (BMJ 1977; Charlton et al. 1973). A strong association between dysuria and the use of soap for perineal toilet was found by Ravnskov (1984). He advocates that women wash their vulva with water alone. Buckley et al. (1978) showed that a small number of organisms may enter the urethra and bladder during coitus. In women in whom the introitus is colonised with coliform organisms, this may lead to urethral infection (Stamey and Sexton 1975). Early voiding after sexual intercourse in these susceptible women may help prevent infection. Potassium citrate mixture taken orally may alleviate symptoms to a variable extent (Maskell et al. 1983). These general measures are all easy to explain to the patient and simple for her to carry out.

Antibiotics

The use of antimicrobial agents is based on the premise that the pyuric patient may have an infectious cause for her symptom complex despite the failure (by definition) to isolate organisms from fractional urines and urethral swabs.

One reason for this failure is that organisms may be present intermittently. Repeated urine culture of patients with initial abacteriuria revealed that 58% of patients developed urinary infection during a 9-month follow-up period (O'Grady et al. 1970). Recovery of introital enterobacteria was higher in patients when symptomatic than when symptom free, thus linking carriage of faecal organisms to urinary infection. However, in this study organisms were also isolated at the introitus in 23% of normal asymptomatic control women, a figure similar to that observed by Stamey and Sexton (1975).

Symptomatic infection of the urethra and para-urethral glands with fastidious organisms (lactobacilli, streptococcus and corynebacterium species) was described by Maskell and co-workers (Maskell 1979, 1983). Sixty-six per cent of their cases showed pyuria, but the rest remained apyuric. The role of lactobacilli, however, has been questioned by other workers (see p. 87).

Stamm et al. (1981) in a double-blind study prescribed doxycycline for both apyuric and pyuric patients, and in this series 11 out of 19 pyuric cases were associated with infection by *Chlamydia trachomatis*. Symptoms and pyuria resolved in the pyuric group including the eight patients without evidence of *Chlamydia* but no beneficial effect could be ascribed to antibiotic therapy in the patients with the acellular 'true' form of the urethral syndrome. These observations support the view expressed by O'Grady et al. (1973) that pyuria occurs in response to a pathological process even if the specific reason cannot be identified at the time of the examination.

Doxycycline is considered to be the initial treatment of choice for patients with the pyuric variant of the urethral syndrome (Stamm et al. 1981). If symptomatic improvement is not recorded or if drug-induced nausea is a problem, erythromycin may be indicated and this agent is also effective against lactobacilli. The use of antibiotics may, however, itself upset the balance of commensal flora and predispose to gram-negative infection (Maskell et al. 1983). In general, antibiotics should be discouraged in patients with apyuria as side-effects such as overgrowth of yeasts and other opportunistic infections may occur (Stamm et al. 1981). This does not seem to be a problem, however, with low-dose treatment and many clinicians are prepared to prescribe erythromycin to apyuric patients in the hope that fastidious organisms might be responsible for symptoms (Maskell et al. 1979).

Pharmacological and Surgical Treatment for the Urethral Syndrome

Urethral hypersensitivity is frequently a feature of the urethral syndrome (Kieswetter 1977; Powell and Feneley 1980) and is often associated with elevated pressures measured during urethral profilometry (see p. 108; Powell et al. 1981). Urethral spasm may theoretically result from increased tension of smooth as well as striated muscle related to the urethra or pelvic floor. In this context phenoxybenzamine decreases urethral pressure by alpha adrenergic blockade of smooth muscle and has been found to facilitate bladder emptying in patients with neurogenic bladder dysfunction (Stanton 1978). Its use has not, however, been evaluated in the urethral syndrome, largely because the side-effects of hypotension and tachycardia are unacceptable in young active women.

Oestrogens and progestagens are known to increase the sensitivity of alpha and beta adrenergic receptors found in both the intrinsic smooth musculature and the vascular bed of the urethral wall (Van Geelen et al. 1981). A decrease in urethral closure pressure was noted in 60% of post-menopausal stress-incontinent women treated with a progesterone derivative causing exacerbation of incontinence (Caine and Raz 1975). Progestagens might possibly be used, therefore, to lower abnormally high urethral closure pressure in continent women.

Kaplan et al. (1980) utilised the known relaxant effect of diazepam therapy on the periurethral striated musculature to treat patients with urethral 'spasm' and reported a complete resolution of symptoms in all six patients after short-term follow-up. O'Boyle and Parsons (1979) considered that bromocriptine might exert an effect on bladder sensation but no therapeutic advantage could be identified for the drug in a double-blind crossover trial of 14 patients with primary sensory urgency. In summary, pharmacological treatment of the urethral syndrome is at an early stage of development and in general is not of practical assistance in the majority of patients suffering from the disorder.

Urethral dilatation may by contrast offer some, albeit temporary, relief to the patient with the urethral syndrome (Roberts and Smith 1968). Dilatation may act either by relieving urethral spasm or by disrupting intramural nerve fibres responsible for the hypersensitive state. Hence it is not possible to determine whether the benefit obtained from urethral dilatation is due to an effect on afferent (urethral hypersensitive state) or efferent (periurethral muscle spasm) target sites.

Dilatation may be performed either under local anaesthesia with lignocaine gel, or under general anaesthesia using graded dilators or an Otis urethrotome without the blade. Some workers routinely perform dilatation under general anaesthesia and prefer the urethrotome to the passage of graduated sounds (Smith 1981). Postoperatively, however, complications of haematuria and temporary incontinence may occur and urethral stenosis may develop in a proportion of cases.

Alternative Surgical Techniques

Symptoms of hesitancy, poor stream and incomplete emptying, which are particularly common in abacteriuric patients (Rees et al. 1976), have led to the belief that outflow obstruction is an important cause of the urethral syndrome. However, studies reported by Hole (1972) and Rees et al. (1976) (see also p. 109) have shown no evidence of urethral obstruction in the majority of patients though reversible urethral spasm may be present and account for some hesitancy and poor flow (Kaplan et al. 1980; Raz and Smith 1976). Such spasm may disturb the laminar flow of urine (Hinman 1968) and may predispose to eddy formation with consequential increase in the rate of urethral infection (Smith 1979).

Fibro-elastosis of the distal half of the urethrovaginal septum was presumed by Richardson (1969) to be the site of principal obstruction and the technique of urethrolysis was devised to excise this band of tissue between the vagina and mucous membrane of the urethra. Using a slight modification of the Richardson operation Splatt and Weedon (1977, 1982) reported relief of symptoms including an improved urinary flow rate in 28 of 40 patients followed for a 5-year period. These studies failed to take account of bacteriuric and abacteriuric patient groups and urodynamic data were incomplete. However Smith et al. (1981), using a similar technique on patients classified preoperatively by full urodynamic studies, reported symptomatic improvement in 87% of patients with recurrent frequency and dysuria.

Histological examination of tissue removed at this operation demonstrates collagenous replacement of urethral smooth muscle, together with clumping of elastic fibres around the smooth muscle bundles (Splatt and Weedon 1981). The success of the operation may be due to a partial denervation of the hypersensitive urethra (Powell et al. 1981) rather than the division of fibro-elastic material, which may not constitute a urodynamic obstruction to the outflow tract.

Internal Urethrotomy

Internal urethrotomy has been advocated as a treatment for recurrent urinary tract infections (Farrar et al. 1973) but in patients with symptoms of frequency and urgency the results were disappointing and this method of treatment cannot be recommended for patients with the urethral syndrome.

Cryosurgical Techniques

Cryosurgery has been employed in the treatment of the urethral syndrome (Parkes and Boreham 1980). A strip of urethra is frozen to a depth of 2–3 mm in both anterior and posterior planes and over a short follow-up period 33 of 35 patients subjectively experienced good results from the procedure. The authors considered that cryosurgery enjoyed several advantages over conventional urethral dilatation, including less discomfort, no increase in frequency and little urethral haemorrhage. However, recent reports indicate that sensation may recover from cryosurgical procedures over a period of months (Sonnex et al. 1985).

Bladder Retraining

Patients with the true urethral syndrome—namely those with negative VB1 and VB2 urinalysis and no evidence of other disease process—generally respond poorly to the treatment modalities so far described. Antibiotics in the absence of infection and excision of fibrous bands in the absence of obstruction are unlikely to produce a positive result in the majority of patients. A rational approach in such cases is to examine whether psychological or nervous mechanisms could play a part in the patient's symptom complex.

Female patients with recurrent cystitis were studied by psychometric tests (Rees and Farhoumand 1977). Patients with inhibited micturition (flow rate <11 ml/s, detrusor pressure >20 cm water) were found to be similar to psychiatric control patients as regards scores of anxiety and obsessionality. These, and other reports (Carson et al. 1980; Kaplan et al. 1980), are the basis upon which bladder retraining schedules have been developed. Therapy is directed towards the control of sensory urgency or frequency symptoms by voluntary suppression of the abnormal micturition habit (Frewin 1980). The aim is to increase the bladder capacity by progressively prolonging the intervals between micturition. Jarvis (1982) considers that bladder training as a hospital in-patient is necessary although Frewin (1980) prefers treatment to be performed on an out-patient basis.

Both these groups have reported similar success rates, 60% of patients being subjectively free of urinary symptoms after follow-up for 6 months. Additionally, objective improvement in measurements of first desire to void and total cystometric capacity was observed by Jarvis (1982). Figure 14.1 shows typical improvement in frequency and voided volume during in-patient bladder training and the improvement being sustained after discharge from hospital. Holmes et al. (1983), reviewing their results of in-patient bladder retraining over a period of 3 years, noted that the best results were obtained in patients with urge symptoms and a stable bladder (sensory urgency) and few of these patients relapsed during the follow-up period.

Many women with the urethral syndrome report that their symptoms are made worse by stress and anxiety. Hypnotherapy has been successful in patients with detrusor instability although a 2-year review showed some relapse and suggested continuing treatment (Freeman and Baxby 1982; Freeman and Guthrie 1985). Both hypnotherapy and psychotherapy have also been used with

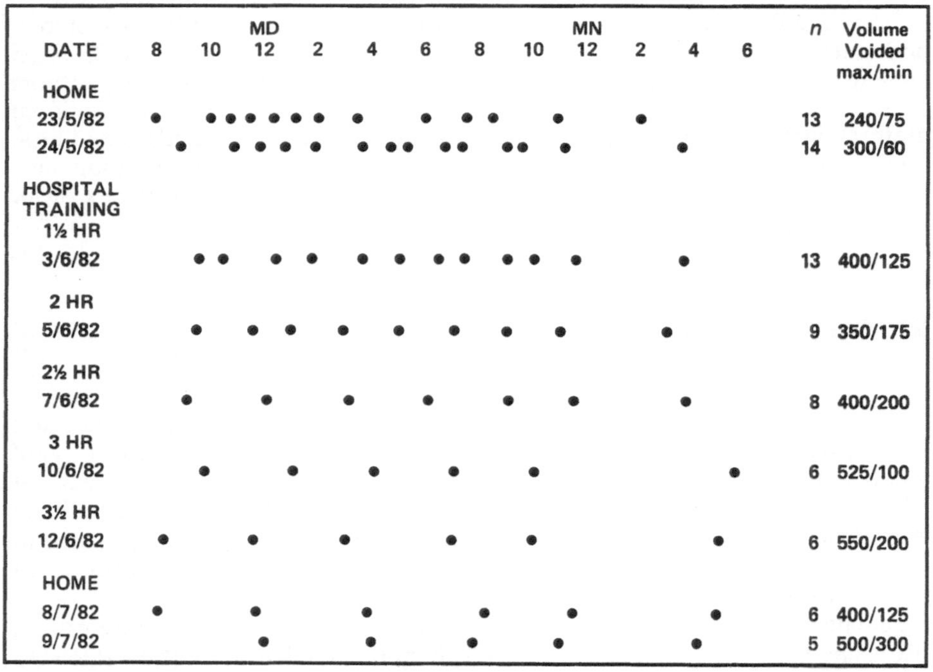

DATE	8	10	MD 12	2	4	6	8	10	MN 12	2	4	6	*n*	Volume Voided max/min
HOME														
23/5/82	•	••	••	••	•	•	••	•		•			13	240/75
24/5/82	•	•	••	•	••	••	•	••	•		•		14	300/60
HOSPITAL TRAINING 1½ HR														
3/6/82		••	•	•	•	••	•	••	•		•		13	400/125
2 HR														
5/6/82		•	••	•		•	•	•	•	•			9	350/175
2½ HR														
7/6/82		•	•		•	•		•	•		•		8	400/200
3 HR														
10/6/82		•		•	•		•	•				•	6	525/100
3½ HR														
12/6/82	•		•		•	•		•			•		6	550/200
HOME														
8/7/82	•		•		•		•		•		•		6	400/125
9/7/82			•		•		•	•			•		5	500/300

Fig. 14.1. Bladder retraining schedule, patient with apyuric urethral syndrome. Patient retraining decreases frequency and increases voided volumes with improvement being maintained at first follow-up out-patient visit.

Table 14.1. Management of apyuric urethral syndrome (St. Mary's Hospital, Manchester)

Initial visit		
Diagnosis:	History (symptoms longer than 6 months) Physical and bacteriological examination Urodynamic assessment: stable bladder high urethral closure pressure Cystourethroscopy	
Treatment:	General hygiene measures Low dose antibiotic, e.g. trimethoprim 100 mg nocte for 2 months Advice regarding out-patient bladder retraining (increase minimum hold)	
Review at 2 months		
Asymptomatic *or*	Improved but still symptomatic or no improvement	
↓	↓	
No treatment	Repeat above management Urethral dilatation under local anaesthesia	
Review at 4 months		
Asymptomatic *or*	Not improved	
↓	↓	
Discharge	Repeat urethral dilatation under local anaesthesia If spasm felt, consider dilatation under general anaesthesia Change antibiotic, e.g. erythromycin 250 mg nocte	
Review at 6 months		
Asymptomatic *or*	Not improved	
↓	↓	
Discharge	Review history: Main problems: Dysuria/frequency Consider urethrolysis	 Main problems: Urgency/frequency In-patient bladder retraining

good effect in the irritable bowel syndrome (Whorwell et al. 1984) and these avenues of treatment could be applied to the urethral syndrome.

Given the lack of organic pathology in these patients, the concept of psychological bladder retraining (Table 14.1) appears to offer a reasonable chance of therapeutic success without the morbidity associated with unnecessary surgical procedures.

References

Asscher AW (1978) Use of antibiotics. Management of frequency and dysuria. Br Med J I:1531–1533

BMJ (1977) The urethral syndrome. Br Med J II:593–594

Buckley RM, McGuckin M, MacGregor RR (1978) Urine bacterial counts after sexual intercourse. N Engl J Med 298:321–324

Caine M, Raz S (1975) Some clinical implications of adrenergic receptors in the urinary tract. Arch Surg 110:247–250

Carson CC, Segura JW, Osborne DM (1980) Evaluation and treatment of the female urethral syndrome. J Urol 124:609–610

Charlton CAC, Cattell WR, Canti G, Grottick J, O'Grady FW (1973) The non urethral syndrome. In: Brumfitt W, Asscher AW (eds) Urinary tract infection. Oxford University Press, Oxford, pp 173–177

Farrar DJ, Green NA, Ashken MH (1973) An evaluation of Otis urethrotomy in female patients with recurrent urinary tract infections. Br J Urol 45:610–615

Freeman RM, Baxby K (1982) Hypnotherapy for incontinence caused by the unstable detrusor. Br Med J 284:1831–1834

Freeman RM, Guthrie KA (1985) Hypnotherapy for the unstable detrusor: a two year review. Br Med J 290:286

Frewin WK (1980) The management of urgency and frequency of micturition. Br J Urol 52:367–369

Hinman F (1968) Bacterial elimination. J Urol 99:811

Hole R (1972) The calibre of the adult urethra. Br J Urol 44:68–70

Holmes DM, Stone AR, Bary PR, Richards CJ, Stephenson TP (1983) Bladder training—3 years on. Br J Urol 55:660–664

Jarvis GJ (1982) The management of urinary incontinence due to primary vesical sensory urgency by bladder drill. Br J Urol 54:374–376

Kaplan WE, Firlit CF, Schoenberg HW (1980) The female urethral syndrome: external sphincter spasm as etiology. J Urol 124:48–49

Kiesswetter H (1977) Mucosal sensory threshold of the urinary bladder and urethra measured electrically. Urol Int 32:437–448

Maskell R, Pead L, Allen J (1979) The puzzle of "urethral syndrome": a possible answer? Lancet I:1058–1059

Maskell R, Pead L, Sanderson RA (1983) Fastidious bacteria and the urethral syndrome: A 2-year clinical and bacteriological study of 51 women. Lancet II:1277–1280

O'Boyle PJ, Parsons KF (1979) Primary vesical sensory urgency: A clinical trial of bromocriptine. Br J Urol 51:200–203

O'Grady FW, Richards B, McSherry MA, O'Farrell SM, Cattell WR (1970) Introital enterobacteria, urinary infection and the urethral syndrome. Lancet II:1208–1210

O'Grady FW, Charlton CAC, Fry IK, McSherry A, Cattell WR (1973) Natural history of intractable 'cystitis' in women referred to a special clinic. In: Brumfitt W, Asscher AW (eds) Urinary tract infection. Oxford University Press, Oxford, pp 81–91

Parkes AC, Boreham P (1980) Cryosurgery for the urethral syndrome: prelimary communication. J R Soc Med 73:428–430

Powell PH, Feneley RCL (1980) The role of urethral sensation in clinical urology. Br J Urol 52:539–541

Powell PH, George NJR, Smith PJB, Feneley RCL (1981) The hypersensitive female urethra—A cuase of recurrent frequency and dysuria. Paper presented at XIth Meeting of the International Continence Society

Ravnskov U (1984) Soap is the major cause of dysuria. Lancet I:1027–1028

Raz S, Smith RB (1976) External sphincter spasticity syndrome in female patients. J Urol 115: 443–446

Rees DLP, Farhoumand N (1977) Psychiatric aspects of recurrent cystitis in women. Br J Urol 49:651–658

Rees DLP, Whitfield HN, Islam AKMS, Doyle PT, Mayo ME, Wickham JEA (1976) Urodynamic findings in adult females with frequency and dysuria. Br J Urol 47:853–860

Richardson FH (1969) External urethroplasty in women: Technique and clinic evaluation. J Urol 101:709–723

Roberts M, Smith P (1968) Non-malignant obstruction of the female urethra. Br J Urol 41:694

Smith PJB (1979) The management of the urethral syndrome. Br J Hosp Med 22:578–587

Smith PJB (1981) The urethral syndrome. Clin Obstet Gynaecol 8:161

Smith PJB, Powell PH, George NJR, Kirk D (1981) Urethrolysis in the management of females with recurrent frequency and dysuria. Br J Urol 53:634–636

Sonnex TS, Jones RL, Weddell AG, Dawber RPR (1985) Long term effects of cryosurgery on cutaneous sensation. Br Med J 290:188–190

Splatt AJ, Weedon D (1977) The urethral syndrome: Experience with the Richardson urethroplasty. Br J Urol 49:173–176

Splatt AJ, Weedon D (1981) The urethral syndrome: Morphological studies. Br J Urol 53:263–265

Splatt AJ, Weedon D (1982) The urethral syndrome: Experience with the Richardson urethroplasty. A review after 5 years. Br J Urol 54:566

Stamey TA, Sexton CC (1975) The role of vaginal colonization with enterobacteriaceae in recurrent urinary infections. J Urol 113:214–217

Stamm WE, Wagner KF, Ansel R, Alexander ER, Turck M, Counts GW, Holmes KK (1980) Causes of the acute urethral syndrome in women. N Engl J Med 303:409–415

Stamm WE, Running K, McKevitt M, Counts GW, Turck M, Holmes KK (1981) Treatment of the acute urethral syndrome. N Engl J Med 304:956–958

Stanton SL (1978) Diseases of the urinary system. Drugs acting on the bladder and urethra. Br Med J I:1607

Whorwell PJ, Prior A, Faragher EB (1984) Controlled trial of hypnotherapy in the treatment of severe refractory irritable-bowel syndrome. Lancet II:1232

Van Geelen JM, Doesburg WH, Thomas CMG, Martin CB (1981) Urodynamic studies in the normal menstrual cycle: The relationship between hormonal changes during the menstrual cycle and the urethral pressure profile. Am J Obstet Gynecol 141:384

Section 4

Prostatodynia

Chapter 15

Inflammatory Prostatic Disease

P.J.C. Brooman

Introduction

Male patients who present with unexplained symptoms of perigenital pain, irritable micturition and sexual dysfunction are frequently diagnosed as suffering from prostatitis. This clinical diagnosis usually heralds a therapeutic onslaught with antibiotics which, although sometimes successful, is often met by a frustrating recurrence or persistence of symptoms, to the increasing disillusionment of both patient and practitioner.

The vague symptoms of this disorder and the lack of physical signs on examination lead inevitably to the consideration of a large number of possible diagnoses (Table 15.1), many of which are unrelated to prostatic pathology. The kidneys, ureters and bladder all share a common segmental autonomic innervation with the prostate, and thus pain emanating from any one of these sites may have the same distribution as prostatic pain (Blacklock 1978). The symptoms of osteitis pubis (Buck et al. 1982) and diverticulitis (Smart et al. 1976) can easily be mistaken for those of prostatic origin. In one recent case the first intimation of the correct diagnosis was the development of a vesicocolic fistula from a pericolic abscess in a young man complaining of persistent 'prostatic' pain.

The lack of a generally accepted definition for prostatitis has been identified by Stamey as one of the major causes of confusion amongst clinicians interested in this disorder, since both diagnostic criteria and pathophysiological changes remain poorly understood (Stamey 1981).

In an attempt to rationalise the prevailing confusion, four categories of benign prostatic disease based upon the analysis of prostatic fluid have been proposed (Drach et al. 1978). The four categories are:

1. Acute bacterial prostatitis
2. Chronic bacterial prostatitis
3. Non-bacterial prostatitis
4. Prostatodynia (pain in the prostate)

The primary task is to determine on the basis of this classification whether or not the patient has prostatitis. This is defined as an inflammatory response within the

Table 15.1. The differential diagnosis of prostatitis

Area	Diagnosis
Urinary tract	Urethritis Urethral stricture Prostate cancer Benign prostatic hyperplasia Cystitis Bladder calculus Detrusor instability Renal/ureteric pathology
Intestinal tract	Anal fissure, Haemorrhoids, Proctitis, Practalgia fugax } 'Anogenital syndrome' Diverticular disease Inflammatory bowel disease Colonic cancer Irritable colon
Other	Osteitis pubis Inguinal, femoral, obturator hernia Prolapsed intervertebral disc Spondylolisthesis Sacroileitis Osteoarthritic hip Autonomic neuropathy Psychiatric disorder

prostate diagnosed by the demonstration of significant numbers of pus cells in the expressed prostatic secretion (EPS). In those patients with a demonstrable inflammatory response, prostatitis may be categorised as bacterial or non-bacterial depending upon the results of bacteriological culture of the EPS. A further sub-division into acute or chronic bacterial prostatitis is made on clinical grounds. Prostatodynia is the name given to patients with symptoms of prostatic pain and no evidence of an inflammatory response in whom all other disorders have been excluded. This terminology has proven successful in both research and clinical practice and is now widely accepted as the basis for rational discussion.

Investigation of the Patient

The first and most important step is to obtain a precise history. There is usually little difficulty in arriving at the correct diagnosis in patients with acute prostatitis. The systemic complaints of these patients consist of malaise, fever and myalgia, which usually precede the development of local inflammatory disturbances of an obstructive or irritative type. The history in cases of chronic or non-bacterial prostatitis may be characterised by periodic exacerbations and remissions whilst some cases of prostatodynia are notable for the relentless persistence of symptoms. It is important to define as accurately as possible the precise nature and location of pain as well as its relationship to voiding, defaecation and coitus. Symptoms of disordered micturition are common and may be related to associated conditions such as urethral stricture or benign prostatic hyperplasia. Urgency and frequency of micturition could be due to an underlying detrusor instability. The presence of blood in the urine should always alert the clinician to the possibility of urinary tract neoplasm. Haemospermia, although usually a less serious sign, also requires additional investigation. Sexual activity is frequently affected, patients complaining of a variety of symptoms, including perineal or penile pain during ejaculation, decreased libido and impotence. Bowel symptoms are particularly important in the differential diagnosis of prostatic discomfort. Perineal pain on defaecation may be caused by prostatitis, especially in a constipated patient. More common causes such as anal fissure should not be overlooked. The identification of factors which exacerbate or relieve prostatic pain is often helpful when attempting to establish the precise diagnosis. Typically, patients with prostatitis notice that their symptoms are worse during exertion, and bed rest in particular may produce marked symptomatic relief.

A full social history is desirable as the patient's occupation may have some bearing on symptoms; long distance drivers in particular may be prone to perineal discomfort. Enquiry must be made of the sexual partner as to whether they have relevant symptoms such as vaginal discharge, dysuria, dyspareunia or pelvic pain. The previous medical history is important, especially if the patient has had surgery to the lower urinary tract or catheterisation, which could be responsible for stricture formation and subsequent development of chronic prostatitis. Most patients with a long history will have received many courses of antibiotic therapy. These must be carefully documented, a note being made of the duration of each course and the clinical response obtained. It is also necessary to establish the time interval between the last course and the date of consultation, as this may affect the interpretation of bacteriological investigations.

The examination of a patient with acute prostatitis usually allows a diagnosis to be reached without difficulty. The patient looks ill and is febrile. There is often suprapubic tenderness and accompanying cystitis, and on rectal examination the prostate feels tense and is exquisitely tender. Scrotal examination may reveal a coexistent epididymitis.

By contrast there are few abnormal findings in the patient with chronic prostatitis and in most cases the prostate feels normal. Areas of induration may be produced by chronic inflammation, calculi, infection or neoplasm. Prostatic tenderness is not a reliable sign of chronic inflammation and in the doubtful case perineal biopsy of the gland should be performed.

The classification of prostatitis suggested by Drach and co-workers depends upon the microscopic examination of the expressed prostatic secretion and urinary bacterial localisation studies, as described by Meares and Stamey (1968). These tests are technically simple and may be performed at the patient's initial visit. Care must be taken during the collection of specimens to ensure that the chances of bacteriological contamination are kept to a minimum. The prepuce, if present, is retracted and the glans penis cleaned with sterile water and dried with a sterile swab. The first 10 ml of urine (voided bladder urine, VB1) is collected in a sterile bottle. The patient is then instructed to continue voiding for a further

150 ml, after which a second bottle is inserted into the stream to collect 10 ml of the mid-stream urine sample (VB2). After the collection the patient stops voiding and following an interval of 30 min prostatic massage is performed. The expressed prostatic secretion (EPS) is collected in a sterile glass petri dish. The first 10 ml of urine voided after prostatic massage (VB3) may provide further evidence of infection localised within the prostate. The various fractional urine specimens and the EPS are plated out on to blood and chocolate agar plates using a 10 μl loop so that comparison of bacterial colony counts can be made. Each specimen is examined microscopically and the number of pus cells per high power field recorded.

Diagnostic Significance of Expressed Prostatic Secretion

Examination of the EPS is central to establishing the diagnosis of prostatitis. Authors differ as to the number of pus cells per high power field necessary to make the diagnosis (Anderson and Weller 1979; Thin and Simmons 1983). Indeed, some workers have suggested that pus cells in the prostatic fluid may be a normal physiological finding (O'Shaugnessy et al. 1956; Jamieson 1967). In general, however, 10 pus cells per high power field is suggestive of prostatitis while 20 pus cells establishes the diagnosis beyond doubt. Clumping of pus cells and a decrease in the number of lecithin granules may also be noted, particularly in acute cases.

Bacterial Studies

In patients with symptoms suggestive of a urethritis, bacterial localisation studies may be successful in indicating the true extent of the inflammation. The VB1 specimen reflects urethral inflammation, whilst the VB3 specimen is an indicator of the state of the prostate. Consequently if the VB2 specimen has a relatively low colony count, and the VB1 count is greater than the VB3 specimen (by a factor of log 1.0), the probable diagnosis is urethritis rather than prostatitis. Conversely, if the VB3 count exceeds the VB1 colony count the diagnosis is prostatitis. Of course, if the patient has a cystitis all the urine colony counts will be uniformly high.

Studies of pH

Further evidence to support the diagnosis of prostatitis may be gained by measuring the pH of the EPS. Blacklock and Beavis (1974) have shown that in patients with prostatitis the EPS, which is normally pH 6.5, becomes alkaline with a pH exceeding 8. This is due to diminished levels of citric acid which persist after the pus cell count has returned to normal (Kavanagh and Derby 1982). Anderson and Fair (1976) have also reported an increase in pH in EPS from patients with documented prostatitis, though the control population in their series had an alkaline mean pH of 7.31. It is possible that an age factor may explain the difference in these observations as ageing is accompanied by a lowering of the citric acid content of expressed prostatic secretion. Further investigation of the patient depends upon the clinical findings and the results of the simple tests outlined above.

General Examination and Investigation of the Prostatitis Patient

It is a sensible precaution to perform a straight abdominal radiograph which includes kidneys, ureters and bladder on all patients. Apart from revealing calcification within the urinary tract and the prostate in particular, it will enable the practitioner to assess the lumbosacral spine, the sacroiliac joints and the pubic symphysis, all of which may produce pain resembling that of prostatic origin.

If the patient has had haematuria or if there is any likelihood of coexistent pathology within the urinary tract, an intravenous urogram is mandatory and the patient will require urethrocystoscopy, which should be covered by an appropriate antibiotic. In patients with chronic prostatitis the finding of minor degrees of urethral stenosis may be significant. Turbulence of urine flow in the region of the prostate can promote reflux of urine to the prostatic ducts, leading to inflammatory change within the gland. In cases in which prostatitis has been excluded and in which detrusor instability or detrusor external sphincter dyssynergia is considered a possibility a full urodynamic assessment should be undertaken. Sigmoidoscopy and barium enema examination are required if the symptoms indicate the possibility of a colonic disorder such as diverticular disease. A bone scan can be helpful in early cases of suspected osteitis pubis, although a plain radiograph is often sufficient to establish this diagnosis (Buck et al. 1982). The diagnosis of prostatodynia can be made only when all these possibilities have been eliminated.

Aetiology of Prostatitis

Bacterial Considerations

Common urinary pathogens, including *E. coli*, enterococci, *Proteus* and *Klebsiella*, may cause acute or chronic bacterial prostatitis, although the role of the gram positive bacteria, particularly *Staphylococcus albus*, is more controversial. Using expressed prostatic secretion Drach (1974) found *Staph. albus* in 37%, streptococci in 21% and diphtheroids in 12% of 105 patients with chronic prostatitis. Although these organisms are common urethral contaminants, their isolation was considered to be significant on the basis that the colony counts obtained in the EPS and VB3 aliquots were at least double those found in the VB1 and VB2 specimens. Furthermore, culture of tissue resected from the periurethral glands grew the same organisms and in two cases staphylococcal septicaemia occurred.

Stamey (1981) criticised these findings, suggesting that there should be at least a ten-fold increase in the colony counts for a positive diagnosis to be achieved and that resected tissue could be contaminated by urethral commensals at the time of removal. However, support for the pathogenicity of staphylococci has been provided by Riedasch et al. (1977), who described an immunofluorescent technique for detecting antibody coating of bacteria in the EPS of patients with prostatitis. In five patients with isolates of *Staph. albus*, antibody coating was demonstrated, confirming the presence of an immune response to this pathogen.

Anatomical and Physiological Factors

The role of anatomical and physiological factors in the aetiology of bacterial prostatitis is less controversial. McNeal (1968) observed that the peripheral zone of the prostate is more frequently involved in chronic inflammation than the remainder of the gland. The ducts draining the peripheral zone open into the urethra at the level of the verumontanum and often run at right angles to the direction of urine flow (Blacklock 1974). In contrast, the ducts of the central zone enter the urethra parallel to the direction of urine flow. This anatomical arrangement tends therefore to promote reflux of urine into the peripheral zone ducts during micturition.

Buck (1975) investigated voiding patterns in patients with prostatitis. Electromyographic studies of the external sphincter revealed evidence of incomplete relaxation during micturition. The turbulence and probable intraprostatic reflux produced by this mechanism could quite easily result in the spread of infection to the prostate.

Kirby et al. (1982) have conclusively demonstrated intraprostatic reflux in a series of elegant studies. They injected Indian ink into the bladders of cadavers, into the bladders of patients with outflow tract obstruction who were later submitted to prostatectomy, and into the bladders of patients with non-bacterial prostatitis. In 70% of the patients with outflow obstruction prostatectomy revealed dye in the peripheral part of the gland. All the patients with prostatitis were found to have macrophages laden with carbon particles on subsequent examination of their EPS.

Further indirect proof of the presence of intraprostatic reflux has been provided by Sutor and Wooley (1974), who found that up to 50% of prostatic calculi were derived from constituents of urine. There seems little doubt that the anatomical disposition of the peripheral zone ducts is responsible to a large degree for the localisation of chronic inflammation to the peripheral part of the gland. It may also be the case that these ducts, which can become ectatic and which frequently harbour prostatic calculi, are responsible for the maintenance of a chronic inflammation. It is possible that bacteria may persist within prostatic stones much as they do in renal struvite calculi (Stamey and Nemoy 1971). Radiological examination of the prostate seldom reveals prostatic calcification but the recently developed technique of rectal ultrasound is able to identify calcification accurately in 80% of patients (Brooman et al. 1981).

Importance of Zinc Concentration

Anderson and Fair (1976) have reported a significant decrease in the concentration of zinc in the EPS of patients with chronic prostatitis. They have shown convincingly that zinc is responsible for the antibacterial activity of prostatic secretion. Zinc is concentrated principally in the peripheral zone of the gland (Kerr et al. 1960) and its secretion appears to be under hormonal control (Blacklock 1976). Hence a change in either hormonal levels or in the ability of the prostatic epithelium to respond to hormonal stimuli could produce a decrease in zinc content of the EPS with consequent enhancement of the risk of infection.

Aetiology of Non-bacterial Prostatitis

The aetiology of non-bacterial prostatitis remains unclear although advances have recently been made in the understanding of this perplexing condition. Possible causes for a purulent EPS secretion yet sterile bacterial culture are listed in Table 15.2. Of particular importance from a practical viewpoint is the patient's recent exposure to antibiotics. It is essential before a diagnosis of non-bacterial prostatitis is made that all antibiotic therapy is stopped for at least one month before bacteriological culture of the EPS is performed. The possibility that viral infection is of aetiological importance has been suggested but there is scant evidence to support this supposition. In a recent study herpes virus and cytomegalovirus have been isolated from prostatic secretion in only 2 of 71 patients at the University Hospital of South Manchester over the past 4 years, and the experience of other authors suggests a similarly low frequency of positive isolates (Gordon et al. 1972). Anaerobic bacterial infections, *Neisseria*

Table 15.2. Possible causes of non-bacterial prostatitis—purulent expressed prostatic secretion with sterile bacteriological culture

1. Previous antibiotics
2. Viral infection
3. *Ureaplasma urealyticum*
4. Anaerobic bacteria
5. *Neisseria*
6. Chemical—urine reflux
   —prostaglandins
7. Autoimmune
8. *Chlamydia trachomatis*

and fungi have likewise been excluded as a cause for this condition by appropriate microbiological techniques (Nielsen and Justesen 1974).

Ureaplasma urealyticum has been proposed as a possible cause for non-bacterial prostatitis (Peters et al. 1983). Other workers (Meares 1973; Thin and Simmons 1983) have been unable to confirm this suggestion. *Ureaplasma* is frequently found as a commensal in the urethra of normal males, which makes its pathogenic significance difficult to evaluate (Viarengo et al. 1980).

It is possible that the mechanisms which tend to produce intraprostatic reflux of urine could lead to a sterile 'chemical' prostatitis. Under these conditions prostaglandins from the seminal vesicles may be important in the mediation of an inflammatory response.

One further possibility is an autoimmune process, induced by the extravasation of prostatic secretion into the stroma. It has been shown that the levels of IgA, IgG and IgM are elevated in these patients, presumably as the result of an antigenic stimulus (Gray et al. 1974). A similar response occurs in patients with bacterial prostatitis which returns to normal with successful antibiotic therapy. In patients with non-bacterial prostatitis the elevated levels often persist, indicating a continuation of the antigenic stimulus.

The Role of *Chlamydia trachomatis*

The most important factor in the aetiology of non-bacterial prostatitis is the possible role played by the obligatory intracellular organism *Chlamydia trachomatis*. Isolation rates of approximately 50% for *Chlamydia trachomatis* have been reported in cases of non-gonococcal urethritis (Perroud and Miedzybrodzka 1978; Oriel et al. 1976). Berger et al. (1978) have demonstrated chlamydial infections in 11 of 23 patients with acute epididymitis. Excluding 10 patients over 35 years of age, of whom most had *E. coli* infections, the chlamydial infection rate was 85%, with positive epididymal aspirates in five out of six cases. Similar results have been reported by Scheibel et al. (1983). It is likely that most patients with epididymitis have a concomitant urethritis and prostatitis and it is therefore probable that *Chlamydia* is the causative organism in non-bacterial prostatitis. Bruce et al. (1981) found an incidence of chlamydial infection in 56% of 70 patients with a clinical diagnosis of chronic prostatitis, but unfortunately the diagnosis in these cases was not based on microscopy of the EPS. Mardh et al. (1978) examined 53 patients with chronic prostatitis. Only one positive chlamydial isolate was obtained from the culture of urethral swabs, with no positive isolates in 28 specimens of EPS.

In most series isolates from prostatic secretion have been rare and until recently none have been reported in the absence of a positive urethral isolate. In a recent study at the University Hospital of South Manchester the diagnosis of non-bacterial prostatitis was made by microscopy and biochemical examination of the EPS in addition to analysis of fractional urine samples. Cultures to isolate *Chlamydia trachomatis* were prepared from the urethra both before and after prostatic massage. A further specimen of EPS together with serum samples were subjected to specific immunoglobulin screening tests. A total of 35 patients fulfilled the above criteria for entry into the study and the age range was between 19 and 66 years, with a mean of 35.5 years. They presented with various symptoms which were primarily irritative in 19 cases, obstructive in 3 cases, and associated with pelvic pain in the remaining 13. The pH of EPS ranged between 6.8 and 8.2 with a mean of 7.3.

Positive urethral isolates of *Chlamydia trachomatis* were obtained in nine patients, four of whom also had positive isolates in their EPS. (The inclusion count in the EPS was, however, lower than that obtained in the urethra by a factor of 30.) Three patients with positive urethral isolates also had IgA specific against *Chlamydia* in their EPS. All nine patients with positive urethral isolates had strongly positive IgG titres in their serum. Although most of these patients presented with primarily irritative symptoms, three cases presented with pelvic pain.

In order to establish whether the positive EPS isolates were genuine, direct needle aspiration of the prostate was attempted in four cases. In one of these aspirates a positive culture was obtained, thus demonstrating that *Chlamydia trachomatis* can exist in prostatic tissue. A further four patients with negative isolates in this study showed strong serological evidence of recent chlamydial infection. Two cases showed a rising antibody titre (×4) and one showed seroconversion. Three of these cases had demonstrable chlamydial-specific IgA in the EPS, evidence of an antibody response to this organism within the prostate.

Hence these data suggest that *Chlamydia trachomatis* may be an aetiological factor in at least one third of patients with non-bacterial prostatitis. Following a 1-month course of treatment, which commonly consisted of either minocycline or erythromycin stearate, all cultures became negative, and the IgG serum antibody level gradually declined to remain at 1:32 over a period of 12 months. The IgA level within the EPS became negative, except in one patient whose symptoms persisted. This case was complicated by a history of genital herpes which may have been in part responsible for the patient's symptoms.

Confirmation that *Chlamydia trachomatis* may be isolated from prostatic fluid has recently been reported by Goh et al. (1983). These workers described two cases with positive EPS isolates who, surprisingly, had no evidence of a urethritis. Both patients had symptoms suggestive of Reiter's syndrome and it is possible that the chlamydial infection may have been implicated in the pathogenesis of the disorder. Ballard et al. (1979) reported a patient with chronic non-bacterial prostatitis who demonstrated a vigorous reaction to skin testing with a strain of *Chlamydia trachomatis*. He regarded this as evidence of a delayed hypersensitivity type of reaction in response to a chlamydial antigenic stimulus. The patient responded to a long course of antibiotic treatment over a period of 5 months. This interesting hypothesis has yet to be confirmed in a larger series of patients.

Chlamydia trachomatis and Cross-reactivity with Frei Antigen

The incidence of positive Frei test reported by King et al. (1956) in a survey of patients attending a venereal clinic was 18.4%, but in only 2% was the diagnosis of lymphogranuloma venereum confirmed by a complement fixation test, although a larger number of patients showed complement-fixing antibodies in the blood. These results were interpreted as indicating an appreciable incidence of undiagnosed lymphogranuloma venereum in the clinic population. In retrospect, a more likely conclusion might be that the positive tests were the result of unsuspected infection with *Chlamydia trachomatis*. If this finding is confirmed by further prospective study, a modified Frei test could become useful as a relatively simple method of picking up cases of chlamydial infection.

Management of Patients with Prostatitis

Acute Bacterial Prostatitis

In the initial acute phase the patient must rest in bed. Relaxation of the pelvic floor muscles is of paramount importance if the symptom complex is to resolve within the shortest possible time. Antibiotic treatment is commenced after the necessary specimens have been collected, so that if necessary therapy can be modified at a later date when the results of sensitivity tests are available. Antibiotics which are minimally ionised penetrate prostatic tissue more easily than acidic antibiotics, which are ionised to a greater degree within plasma. An understanding of these aspects of membrane transport determines that Septrin or trimethoprim is commonly the initial treatment of choice. Other antibiotics which are frequently prescribed are erythromycin stearate and minocycline, which are both active against staphylococci. Treatment is usually continued for a period of 1 month, after which the patient is re-examined to ensure that the prostatitis has cleared.

Chronic Bacterial Prostatitis

In these patients a complete urological evaluation is necessary to demonstrate any factors which might predispose towards recurrent infection; urethral strictures, calculi or anatomical and functional anomalies may be important in this respect. Antibiotic treatment is again based upon bacterial culture and sensitivities, the range of antibiotics described above being appropriate for the condition. Therapy may need to be prolonged for many months to eradicate persistent infection. In some cases, where palpable foci of infection or multiple prostatic calculi are demonstrated, there may be a need for transurethral resection (Blacklock 1974). However, the results of this procedure are disappointing in the majority of these patients.

Non-bacterial Prostatitis

The findings reported above and those of others regarding the likelihood of chlamydial infection in this condition lead to the recommendation of an appropriate antibiotic which should be taken for a period of at least 1 month. Both minocycline and erythromycin have been found to be very effective against this organism. It is particularly important in cases of chlamydial infection to examine and, if necessary, treat, the consort in order to prevent the occurrence of reinfection. In those patients with non-bacterial prostatitis who do not have any evidence of chlamydial infection, and whose serology remains negative, the outlook remains unsatisfactory. The response to further courses of antibiotics is generally poor, as is the response to most other forms of treatment, including steroids and non-steroidal anti-inflammatory agents (Stamey 1981).

Prostatodynia

In this group of patients, who complain of 'prostatic' pain but show no evidence of an inflammatory reaction within the prostate, recognition of the condition is entirely dependent on careful history taking and examination. The diagnosis may only be made after all other possible causes for the symptom complex have been excluded. This is often difficult, particularly as many patients have initially been diagnosed as cases of prostatitis and treated with multiple courses of antibiotics. The essential feature of the diagnosis remains the absence of pus cells in the expressed prostatic secretion. This enigmatic condition will be considered in greater detail elsewhere (p. 139).

The Urinary Tract Infection Clinic

Experience in dealing with cases of prostatitis over a number of years has confirmed the benefits and value of a specialised urinary tract infection clinic. The relatively small number of patients who attend this facility ensure that time is available to obtain a full history and perform a thorough examination. The

Table 15.3. Routine investigation schedule for patient attending prostatitis clinic at University Hospital of South Manchester

1. History	
2. Examination	
VB1+VB2	Colony count+pus cell count
Urethral swab	Chlamydial culture[a]
EPS	pH (Duotest—Machery Nagel & Co.)
	Biochemistry (Zn, citrate, SAP)
	Bacteriological culture (chocolate/blood, agar innoculation 10 μl loop)
	Fungal culture (Sabouraud's medium)
	Chlamydial culture
	Chlamydial IgA
	Electron microscopy (virus particles)
Urethral swab	Chlamydial culture
VB3	Colony count+pus cell count
Blood	Chlamydial Ab titre (IgG, IgM)
	Specific bacterial IgG
3. Plain abdominal radiograph	

[a] Transport medium required

clinic allows a close liaison to be maintained with the Departments of Bacteriology, Virology and Serology for the proper and timely collection of specimens. Table 15.3 shows the routine procedure for the examination of a case of prostatitis. A close relationship with the various laboratories who are best able to advise on the necessary procedures for obtaining specimens and the interpretation of results is clearly desirable and particularly so in the case of *Chlamydia trachomatis*, for which the isolation techniques are laborious and the serological techniques may be open to misinterpretation (Richmond 1979). Skilled nursing personnel are invaluable and may help with the collection, identification and despatch of specimens. They also play an important role in the management of each patient, especially in cases where it is necessary to interview and examine the consort.

References

Anderson RU, Weller C (1979) Prostatic secretion leukocyte studies in non-bacterial prostatitis (prostatosis). J Urol 121:292–294

Anderson RU, Fair WR (1976) Physical and chemical determinations of prostatic secretion in benign hyperplasia, prostatitis and adenocarcinoma. Invest Urol 14:137–140

Ballard RC, Block C, Koornhof HJ, Haitas B (1979) Delayed hypersensitivity to *Chlamydia trachomatis*: Cause of chronic prostatitis? Lancet II:1305–1306

Berger RE, Alexander ER, Monda GD, Ansell J, McCormick G, Holmes KK (1978) *Chlamydia trachomatis* as a cause of acute "idiopathic" epididymitis. N Engl J Med 298:301–304

Blacklock NJ (1974) Anatomical factors in prostatitis. Br J Urol 46:47–54

Blacklock NJ (1976) The anatomy of the prostate. In: Williams DI, Chisholm MGD (eds) Scientific foundations of urology. Heinemann, London, pp 113–125

Blacklock NJ (1978) Prostatic pain. Br J Hosp Med 20:80–81

Blacklock NJ, Beavis JP (1974) The response of prostatic fluid pH in inflammation. Br J Urol 46:537–542

Brooman PJC, Griffiths GJ, Roberts E, Peeling WB, Evans K (1981) Per rectal ultrasound in the investigation of prostatic disease. Clin Radiol 32:669–676

Bruce AW, Chadwick T, Willett WS, O'Shaughnessy M (1981) The role of *Chlamydia* in genito-urinary disease. J Urol 126:625–629

Buck AC (1975) Disorders of micturition in bacterial prostatitis. Proc R Soc Med 68:508–511

Buck AC, Crean DM, Jenkins IL (1982) Osteitis pubis as a mimic of prostatic pain. Br J Urol 54:741–744

Drach GW (1974) Problems in the diagnosis of prostatitis; gram-negative, gram-positive and mixed infections. J Urol 111:630–636

Drach GW, Fair WR, Meares EM, Stamey TA (1978) Classification of benign diseases associated with prostatic pain: prostatitis or prostatodynia? J Urol 120:266

Fair WR, Couch J, Wëhner N (1976) Prostatic antibacterial factor. Identity and significance. Urology 7:169–177

Goh BT, Morgan-Capner P, Lim KS (1983) Isolation of *Chlamydia trachomatis* from prostatic fluid in association with inflammatory joint and eye disease. Br J Vener Dis 59:373–375

Gordon HL, Miller DH, Rawis WE (1972) Viral studies in patients with non-specific prostatourethritis. J Urol 108:299–300

Gray SP, Billings J, Blacklock NJ (1974) Distribution of the immunoglobulins G, A and M in the prostatic fluid of patients with prostatitis. Clin Chim Acta 57:163–169

Jamieson RN (1967) Sexual activity and the variation of white cell content of prostatic secretion. Invest Urol 5:297

Kavanagh JP, Derby C (1982) The interrelationship between acid phosphatase, amino peptidase, diamine oxidase, citric acid, beta glucuronidase, pH and zinc in human prostatic fluid. Int J Androl 5:503–512

Kerr WK, Keresteci AG, Kayoh H (1960) The distribution of zinc within the human prostate. Cancer 13:550–554

King AJ, Barwell CF, Catterall RD (1956) Intradermal tests in the diagnosis of lymphogranuloma venereum. Br J Vener Dis 32:209–216

Kirby RS, Lowe D, Bultitude MI, Shuttleworth KED (1982) Intraprostatic urinary reflux; an aetiological factor in abacterial prostatitis. Br J Urol 54:729–731

Mardh PA, Ripa KT, Colleen S, Treharne JD, Darougar S (1978) Role of *Chlamydia trachomatis* in non-acute prostatitis. Br J Vener Dis 54:330–334

McNeal JE (1968) Regional morphology and pathology of the prostate. Am J Clin Pathol 49:347–357

Meares EM Jr (1973) Bacterial prostatitis vs "prostatosis". A clinical and bacteriological study. JAMA 224:1372–1375

Meares EM Jr, Stamey TA (1968) Bacterial localisation patterns in prostatitis and urethritis. Invest Urol 5:492–518

Nielsen ML, Justesen T (1974) Studies on the pathology of prostatitis. A search for prostatic infections with obligate anaerobes in patients with chronic prostatitis and chronic urethritis. Scand J Urol Nephrol 8:1–6

Oriel JD, Reeve P, Wright JT, Owen J (1976) Chlamydial infection of the male urethra. Br J Vener Dis 52:46–51

O'Shaughnessy EJ, Parrino PS, White JD (1956) Chronic prostatitis—fact or fiction? JAMA 160:540–542

Perroud HM, Miedzybrodzka K (1978) Chlamydial infection of the urethra in men. Br J Vener Dis 54:45–49

Peters M, Polack-Vogelzang A, Debruyne F, Van Der Veen J (1983) Abacterial prostatitis, microbiological data. In: Brunner H, Krause W, Rothauge GF, Weidner W (eds) Chronische Prostatitis. Internationale Arbeitstagung, Bad Nauheim, 1981. Schattauer, Stuttgart New York

Richmond SJ (1979) Immunofluorescence testing for chlamydial antibodies. Lancet II:1016

Riedasch G, Ritz E, Möhring K, Ikinger U (1977) Antibody-coated bacteria in the ejaculate; a possible test for prostatitis. J Urol 118:787–788

Schiebel JH, Anderson JT, Brandenhoff P, Geerdson JP, Bay-Nielson A, Schultz BA, Walter S (1983) *Chlamydia trachomatis* in acute epididymitis. Scand J Urol Nephrol 17:47–50

Smart CJ, Jenkins JD, Lloyd RS (1976) The painful prostate. Br J Urol 47:861–869

Stamey TA (1981) Prostatitis. J R Soc Med 74:22–39

Stamey TA, Nemoy NJ (1971) Surgical, bacteriological and biochemical management of "infection stones". JAMA 215:1470–1476

Sutor DJ, Wooley SE (1974) The crystaline composition of prostatic calculi. Br J Urol 46:533–535

Thin RN, Simmons PD (1983) Chronic bacterial and non-bacterial prostatitis. Br J Urol 55:513–518

Viarengo J, Hebrant F, Piot P (1980) *Ureaplasma urealyticum* in the urethra of healthy men. Br J Vener Dis 56:169–172

Chapter 16

Prostatodynia—Clinical Aspects

D.E. Osborn

Introduction

The diagnosis of prostatitis is frequently given to men who present with symptoms of chronic genital pain and irritative voiding disturbances. Many of these cases will have previously received extensive courses of antibiotics with only sporadic success, leading to disillusionment on the part of both the patient and the clinician. Extensive studies and analysis of both fractional urine samples and expressed prostatic secretion (EPS) by Drach et al. (1978) resulted in the first rational classification of the inflammatory prostatic disorders (for full account see p. 127). 'Prostatodynia' was suggested by these authors as a logical term to describe symptomatic patients with sterile EPS on culture and few (less than 8 per h.p.f.) leucocytes on direct microscopy. Essentially, therefore, patients with prostatodynia have symptoms of longstanding genital pain associated with voiding disturbances, normal fractional urine specimens and sterile cell-free expressed prostatic secretion.

These patients are typically tense, anxious and often highly introverted and in some cases such emotional disturbances may be thought to play a part in the persistence of the symptom complex (Keltikangas-Järvinen et al. 1981). The personality traits common in prostatodynia are not, however, specific to this complaint and similar observations have been reported in patients with such diverse problems as chronic back pain (Sternbach et al. 1973), frozen shoulder (Coventry 1953), abdominal pain (Gomez and Dally 1977) and female pelvic inflammatory disease (Beard et al. 1977; Renaer et al. 1979).

The absence of objective evidence of disease leads to difficulties in the assessment of both the individual case and the response to treatment obtained in groups of patients followed over a period of time. Recent prospective studies, however, have shed some light on the pathophysiological mechanisms of the condition and led to a more complete understanding of the prostatodynia symptom complex (Osborn et al. 1981).

Aetiology of Prostatodynia

The genesis of prostatodynia in most patients is unknown. In some there is an undoubted past episode of acute prostatitis which is followed by longstanding symptoms, despite evidence confirming resolution of the previous infection. Some patients may relate the commencement of their symptoms to an extramarital affair and under these circumstances anxiety may be thought to play a part in the chronicity of the disorder. Segura et al. (1979) reported on association of prostatitis-like symptoms with long-distance driving and suggested that this resulted from a tension myalgia of the pelvic floor occurring in individuals with a tendency to a tense and neurotic personality. It was not clear from this study, however, whether bacterial infection had preceded the development of the patients' symptoms.

Clinical Features

Most patients with prostatodynia are between the ages of 30 and 60. The diagnosis, though never straightforward, is made easier in younger patients by the absence of symptoms attributable to prostatic enlargement which occur in older men. The major symptom of patients with prostatodynia is that of *pain* which is usually described as being centred in the perineum and which varies from a mild ache to a persistent, dull, boring discomfort. The disorder may be present for many years, and attacks, whilst remitting from time to time in the majority of cases, commonly last for several months without relief. The pain is frequently exacerbated by ejaculation and, for some men, this becomes of predominant importance.

Associated discomfort may be experienced in the suprapubic area, penis, testes, epididymides and loins, and in some patients pain radiating from one of these areas may be the principal complaint (Table 16.1).

Symptoms of urinary voiding disturbances have been recorded by several authors and are usually attributed to obstructive dysfunction at bladder neck level, though this is disputed by others (Osborn et al. 1981). Peak urine flow-rate may indeed be reduced in patients with prostatitis (Drach and Binnard 1976) and prostatodynia (Osborn et al. 1981) when compared with normal age-matched

Table 16.1. Somatic and urodynamic symptoms in 37 male patients with prostatodynia. The diagnosis had been established by clinical, bacteriological and urodynamic screening

Somatic symptoms		Urodynamic symptoms	
Perineal pain	76%	Post-micturition dribble	35%
Pain after ejaculation	56%	Hesitancy	26%
Suprapubic discomfort	55%	Persistent urethral sensation	23%
Penile pain	44%	Strain to void	17%
Testicular pain/aches	35%		
Loin pain	17%		

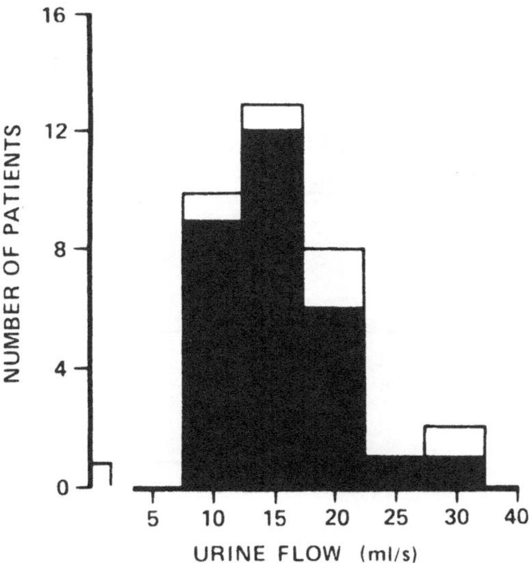

Fig. 16.1. Initial urinary flow rate in 35 patients with prostatodynia. Mean flow rate, 16 ml/s, is low when compared with age-matched controls, but not so low as to lead commonly to a complaint of poor stream. *Open boxes*, flow rate increase after transurethral resection. Little improvement is observed, illustrating the non-obstructive nature of the condition.

controls. However, since the urine flow-rate is commonly greater than 10 ml/s in most patients few make a primary complaint of poor urinary stream (Fig. 16.1). Increased frequency with nocturia is variable, but if excessive should lead to objective assessment by means of a frequency/volume chart (see below, Fig. 16.2). Psychological and psychophysiological aspects of the disorder are described in detail in Chap. 18.

The Anxious Bladder

Occasionally patients are encountered whose lower urinary tract symptoms appear to be merely one facet of a more generalised psychological disorder. The nature of the general complaint and the personality of these patients has led some workers to describe the urological symptom complex as the 'anxious bladder syndrome' (George and Slade 1979).

The majority of patients present in their fourth decade and a significant percentage lead a stressful lifestyle. The urological symptoms often exhibit a marked periodicity similar to that recorded in cases of duodenal ulceration. The implication of this observation was pursued by George and Slade (1979), who found upper gastrointestinal complaints requiring regular antacid therapy to be present in 10 of 16 patients, 5 of whom had previously undergone oral barium studies. All of these tests, however, proved negative. The incidence of dyspepsia in this group of patients was approximately twice that expected even when

IF YOU ARE TO ATTEND FOR AN I.V.P. – THAT IS AN X–RAY OF YOUR KIDNEYS AND BLADDER – DO NOT KEEP ANY RECORD ON THE DATE THAT YOU ATTEND FOR THE X–RAY EXAMINATION.

DAY	TIME / VOLUME DAY TIME (measure volumes in mls, ccs or **fl. oz.**)	TIME / VOLUME NIGHT TIME
1		
2	7.30 16 9.00 4 11.15 – 3.30 – 5.30 5 12.15 15	6am 6
3	7.00/20 8am 4 11am – 1pm – 4pm – 6.20/5 8pm 4 10.30/7	3am /4
4	8am /9 11.00/4 2.15pm 5 5.30 5 8pm 3 10.00/2 11.00/7	6.30/4
5	7.30 am/12 9.00/– 12 midday/– 5pm – 7.00/4 9.15/6 11.30/10	3am / 10
6	7am /21 9.00/2 10.00/– 1pm – 5.00/– 7.30 4 11.45 20	7am 12
7		

Fig. 16.2. Frequency/volume chart in patient aged 35 with prostatodynia. Moderate frequency by day with mild nocturia. This degree of frequency would probably not be a cause for complaint if the patient did not have other symptoms. (1 fl. oz. = 30 ml.).

comparison was made with the 'normal' population resident in ulcer prone areas of the country (Doll and Jones 1951; Weir and Backett 1968). These observations lend weight to the theories suggesting a psychological origin for the urological symptom complex

Frequency of micturition may be severe by day but is unusual at night (Fig. 16.3). Most patients describe the desire to pass urine as a persistent 'nag' or sensation located in the posterior urethral area but this only rarely attains the level of discomfort described by patients with prostatodynia. Pronounced hesitancy is a common complaint and leads in some cases to a characteristic inability to micturate in a public toilet. These patients are apparently unable to initiate micturition whilst in the presence of strangers and prefer to void alone in a cubicle. Some patients have even been unable to urinate in the privacy of their own home if, for example, their children are playing in the proximity of the toilet. This extraordinary symptom, which may be life-long in duration, is usually diagnostic of the anxious bladder syndrome.

Suprapubic bladder pain, noted particularly if micturition is unduly delayed, loin ache and discomfort at the commencement of voiding are less debilitating symptoms described by some patients. The urine flow is commonly intermittent in nature though a Valsalva manoeuvre is often performed in an attempt to diminish hesitancy and enhance the process of voiding.

The diagnosis of an anxious bladder is, therefore, dependent upon the identification of a number of interrelated abnormalities and not on the observation of a particular symptom complex emanating from a single system (Fig. 16.4). However, it may be premature to assume that the multisystem nature of the disorder is conclusive evidence of a psychological aetiology. Poor stream in a young man due to organic bladder neck obstruction may give rise to a considerable degree of anxiety, and a psychological diagnosis is clearly inappropriate in such cases. Hence, the diagnosis of anxious bladder syndrome can only be substantiated with urodynamic studies which are fully described in Chap. 17.

Post-micturition dribble is the most troublesome symptom for many patients with either prostatodynia or the anxious bladder syndrome. The history, combined with urodynamic findings, suggests that in these patients the bladder neck closes prematurely after voiding, isolating urine in the prostatic urethra. This small volume of urine presumably leaks distally following partial relaxation of the striated periurethral muscle of the pelvic floor (Fig. 16.5). Full evaluation of this phenomenon requires video cystometric examination, though this is rarely undertaken in such patients for reasons described elsewhere (p. 34). This hypothesis as to the cause of post-micturition dribbling is supported by the symptomatic relief obtained by the use of the alpha blocking agent phenoxybenzamine, which presumably relaxes the bladder neck and permits orderly milk-back of urine into the bladder.

Examination and Investigation

Examination

Physical examination of patients with prostatodynia or anxious bladder is essentially negative and any abnormality will suggest an alternative diagnosis. Prostatic tenderness on rectal examination is an unreliable sign of prostatitis or prostatodynia as it is present in at least 25% of the normal patient population (Smart et al. 1976). Segura et al. (1979) described an increase in tone of the puborectalis muscle and whilst some have found this sign to be inconsistently present (Osborn et al. 1981), rectal examination is without doubt particularly difficult in anxious bladder patients due to spasm of the pelvic floor muscles.

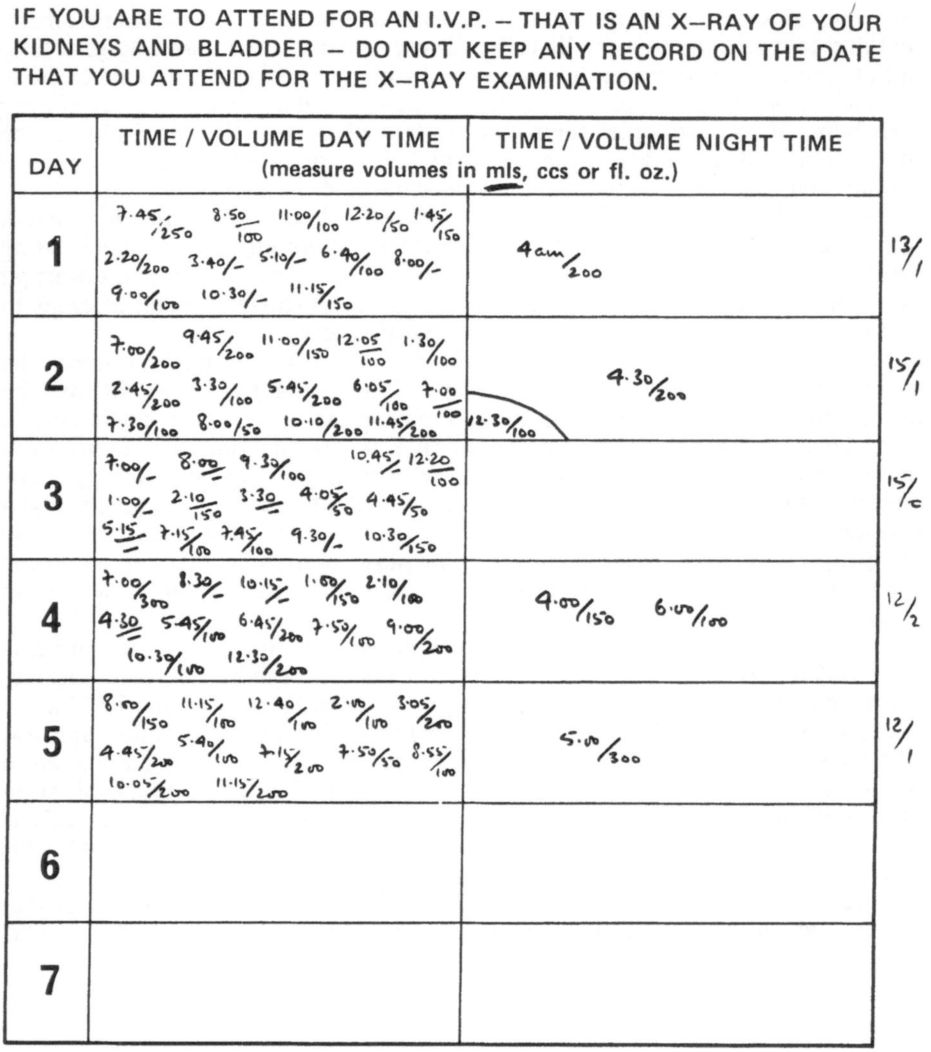

IF YOU ARE TO ATTEND FOR AN I.V.P. – THAT IS AN X–RAY OF YOUR KIDNEYS AND BLADDER – DO NOT KEEP ANY RECORD ON THE DATE THAT YOU ATTEND FOR THE X–RAY EXAMINATION.

DAY	TIME / VOLUME DAY TIME (measure volumes in mls, ccs or fl. oz.)	TIME / VOLUME NIGHT TIME	
1	7.45/250 8.50/100 11.00/100 12.20/50 1.45/150 2.20/200 3.40/– 5.10/– 6.40/100 8.00/– 9.00/100 10.30/– 11.15/150	4am/200	13/1
2	7.00/200 9.45/200 11.00/150 12.05/100 1.30/100 2.45/200 3.30/100 5.45/200 6.05/100 7.00/100 7.30/100 8.00/50 10.10/200 11.45/200	12.30/100 4.30/200	15/1
3	7.00/– 8.00/– 9.30/100 10.45/– 12.20/100 1.00/– 2.10/150 3.30/– 4.05/50 4.45/50 5.15/– 7.15/100 7.45/100 9.30/– 10.30/150		15/0
4	7.00/300 8.30/– 10.15/– 1.00/150 2.10/100 4.30/– 5.45/100 6.45/200 7.50/100 9.00/200 10.30/100 12.30/200	4.00/150 6.00/100	12/2
5	8.00/150 11.15/100 12.40/100 2.00/100 3.05/200 4.45/200 5.40/100 7.15/200 7.50/50 8.55/100 10.05/200 11.15/200	5.00/300	12/1
6			
7			

a

Fig. 16.3. **a** Frequency/volume chart of patient with anxious bladder syndrome. Note the typical features of a 'psychogenic' voiding pattern—little nocturia and the nearly normal volume of the first morning void. **b** Day and night frequency in 16 patients with anxious bladder syndrome. (George and Slade 1979)

Investigation

A full urological investigation is mandatory in patients with a suspected diagnosis of prostatodynia or anxious bladder in order to exclude pathological processes involving the lower urinary tract. Fractional urines (VB1, VB2, VB3), prostatic fluid analysis, serology, blood biochemical profile and intravenous urography are normal in these patients. At cystoscopy the bladder

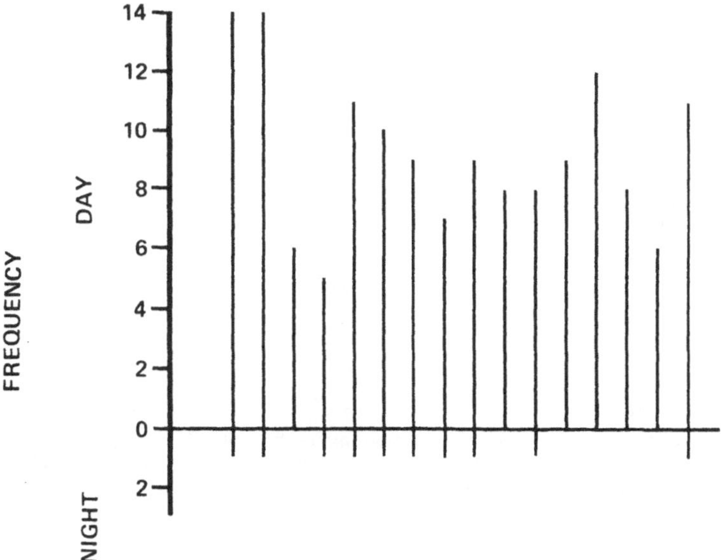

Fig. 16.3b

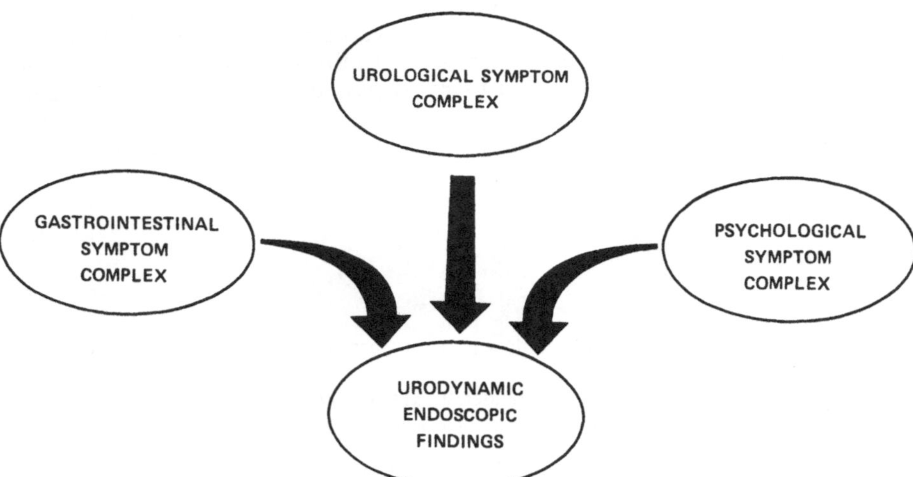

Fig. 16.4. The anxious bladder syndrome. The diagnosis rests on the identification of multisystem abnormalities.

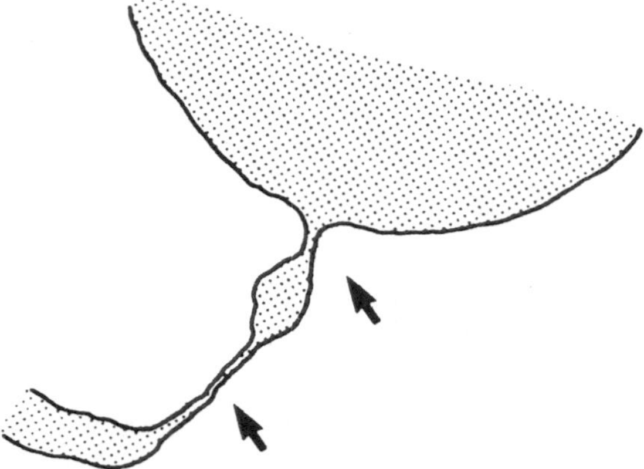

Fig. 16.5. Possible cause of post-micturition dribble in over-anxious patients. *Arrows*, bladder neck and external urethral sphincter zones. Following micturition the bladder neck sphincter may close prematurely, thus preventing milk-back and allowing the small volume of urine 'trapped' within the prostatic urethra to trickle out distally.

appears normal and little or no evidence of bladder neck obstruction is seen. Rigid adherence to the diagnostic criteria is important since once diagnosed as a case of prostatodynia the patient may become insulated from the customary clinical awareness which should particularly apply to patients with longstanding and undiagnosed pain.

Frequency/Volume Charts

The urinary frequency in prostatodynia and the anxious bladder syndrome resembles that found in the female urethral syndrome (Figs. 16.2, 16.3). The voiding interval is related to the perineal or urethral discomfort and at night most patients do not rise more than twice to pass urine. This pattern is quite different from that found in other bladder disorders where frequency is related to a reduced capacity and continues relentlessly both by day and night.

References

Beard RW, Belsey EM, Lieberman BA, Wilkinson JCM (1977) Pelvic pain in women. Am J Obstet Gynecol 128:566–570

Coventry MB (1953) Problem of painful shoulder. JAMA 151:177–185

Doll R, Jones SA (1951) Occupational factors in the aetiology of gastric and duodenal ulcers. Special MRC Report No. 276

Drach GW, Binard W (1976) Disposable peak urinary flowmeter estimates of lower urinary tract obstruction. J Urol 115:175–179

Drach GW, Fair WR, Meares EM, Stamey TA (1978) Classification of benign diseases associated with prostatic pain; prostatitis or prostatodynia? J Urol 120:266

George NJR, Slade N (1979) Hesitancy and poor stream in neurologically normal younger men without outflow obstruction. Br J Urol 51:506–510

Gomez J, Dally P (1977) Psychologically mediated abdominal pain in surgical and medical outpatient clinics. Br Med J I:1451–1453

Keltikangas-Järvinen L, Järvinen H, Lehtonen T (1981) Psychic disturbances in patients with chronic prostatitis. Ann Clin Res 13: 45–49

Osborn DE, George NJR, Rao PN, Barnard RJ, Reading C, Marklow C, Blacklock NJ (1981) Prostatodynia—Physiological characteristics and rational management with muscle relaxants. Br J Urol 53:621–623

Renaer M, Vertommen H, Nijs P, Wagemans L, Hemelrijck TV (1979) Psychological aspects of chronic pelvic pain in women. Am J Obstet Gynecol 134:75–80

Segura JW, Opitz JL, Greene LF (1979) Prostatosis, prostatitis or pelvic floor tension myalgia? J Urol 122:168–169

Smart CJ, Jenkins JD, Lloyd RS (1976) The painful prostate. Br J Urol 47:861–869

Sternbach RA, Wolf SR, Murphy RW, Akeson WH (1973) Aspects of chronic low back pain. Psychosomatics 14:52

Weir RV, Backett EM (1968) Incidence of dyspeptic symptoms in North-East Scotland. Gut 9:75–83

Chapter 17

Prostatodynia and Anxious Bladder—Urodynamic Aspects

N.J.R. George

Introduction

Other than the brief reports by Drach and Binard (1976) and Siroky et al. (1981) there have been no detailed urodynamic studies of patients with prostatodynia. This is surprising as it is often assumed that 'obstruction' is present in these patients and transurethral resection of the prostate (usually with little improvement: Stamey 1981) is often performed.

The importance of good urodynamic technique when examining patients with a tendency to anxiety and introspection has been emphasised in Chap. 4. Patients should initially pass urine in complete privacy and must be instructed not to assist their flow rate by pushing. Urethral pressure profile measurement by the method of Brown and Wickham (1969) is followed by medium fill water cystometry (60 ml/min) and subsequent voiding studies should again be performed with the patient alone in the examination room in order to allow maximum relaxation during micturition (George and Slade 1979).

Using such techniques, Osborn et al. (1981) found a consistent urodynamic pattern in patients with prostatodynia, reflecting careful clinical and bacteriological screening of patients in the clinic prior to referral for urodynamic evaluation. On occasion the presence of irritative voiding disturbances may raise the question as to whether the patient's symptoms are a consequence of unstable bladder contractions and it is known that the diagnosis of bladder instability from symptoms alone presents considerable difficulties in older men. However, the same is not true of their younger counterparts and symptoms of urgency, urge incontinence, and enuresis were significantly related to bladder instability ($P=<0.05$) in 106 men studied between the ages of 20 and 45 years by Abrams et al. (1981). Thus informed history taking in younger men at the time of the initial clinic visit may successfully exclude patients with bladder instability, particularly if uroflowmetry is also performed as part of the screening procedure (George 1985).

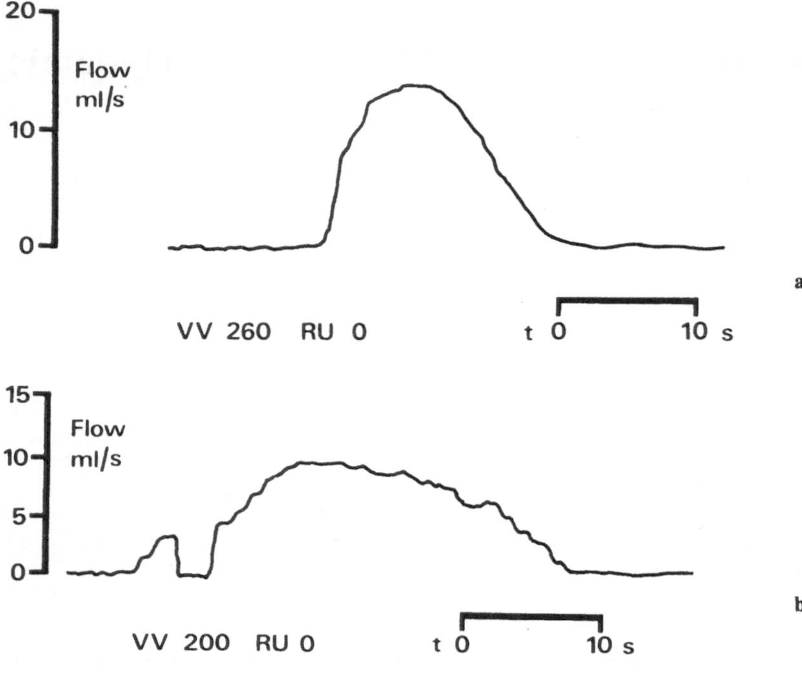

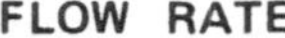

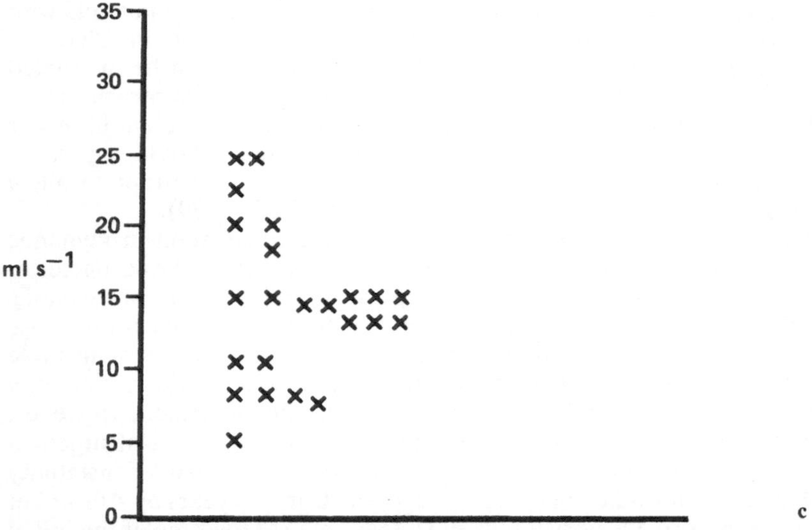

Fig. 17.1. Initial flow rate in prostatodynia for **a** man aged 36, **b** man aged 32. Reasonable voided volumes and relatively normal shape of flow curve. The maximum values are, however, considerably less than those expected of normal men of equivalent age. **c** Initial flow rate in 23 patients with prostatodynia.

Urodynamic Observations

Observations in Prostatodynia

The initial mean maximum urine flow rate in 27 patients (mean age 42 years) with prostatodynia was 16.2 ml/s ± 0.9 SE (Osborn et al. 1981), results comparable to those previously recorded by Drach and Binard (1976) in patients with chronic prostatitis (Fig. 17.1). The mean maximum urethral closure pressure (MUCP) was 121 cm H_2O ± 9.3 SE, a level in excess of that expected for healthy controls of the same age (Fig. 17.2). All cystometric studies in these patients were stable and the mean capacity at the normal desire to micturate was 320 ml. Voiding cystometry demonstrated a mean intrinsic detrusor pressure (Pdet) of 34 cm H_2O ± 2 SE, associated with a mean maximum urine flow rate of 15 ml/s ± 1 SE (Fig. 17.3; Osborn et al. 1981).

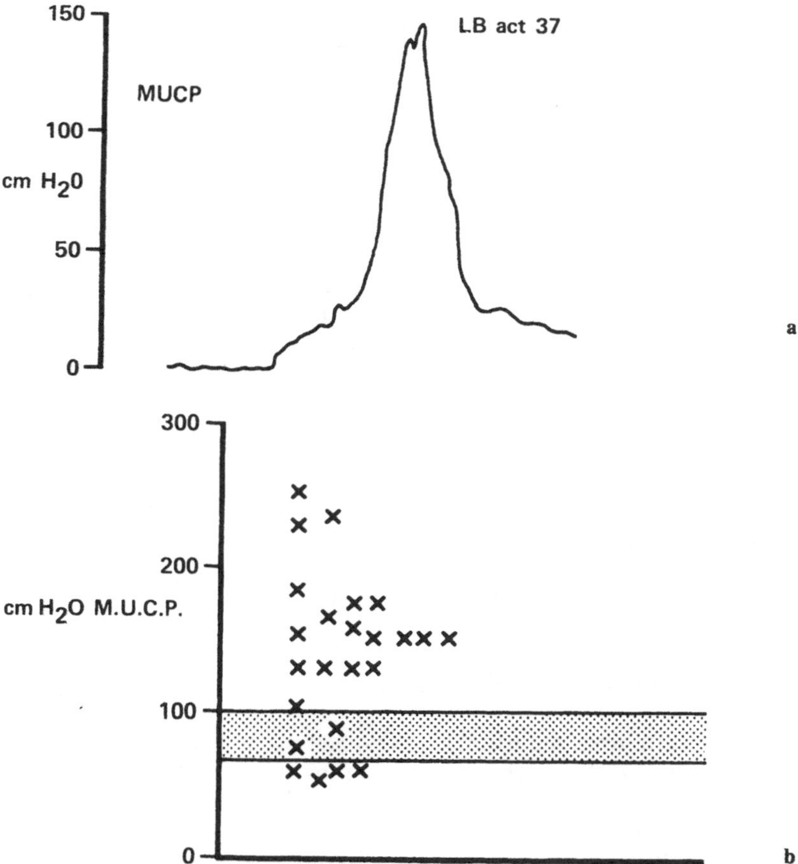

Fig. 17.2. **a** Urethral pressure profile in prostatodynia patient aged 37. **b** Values of maximum closure pressure in 24 patients with prostatodynia. *Stippled area*, normal range. (Abrams et al. 1983)

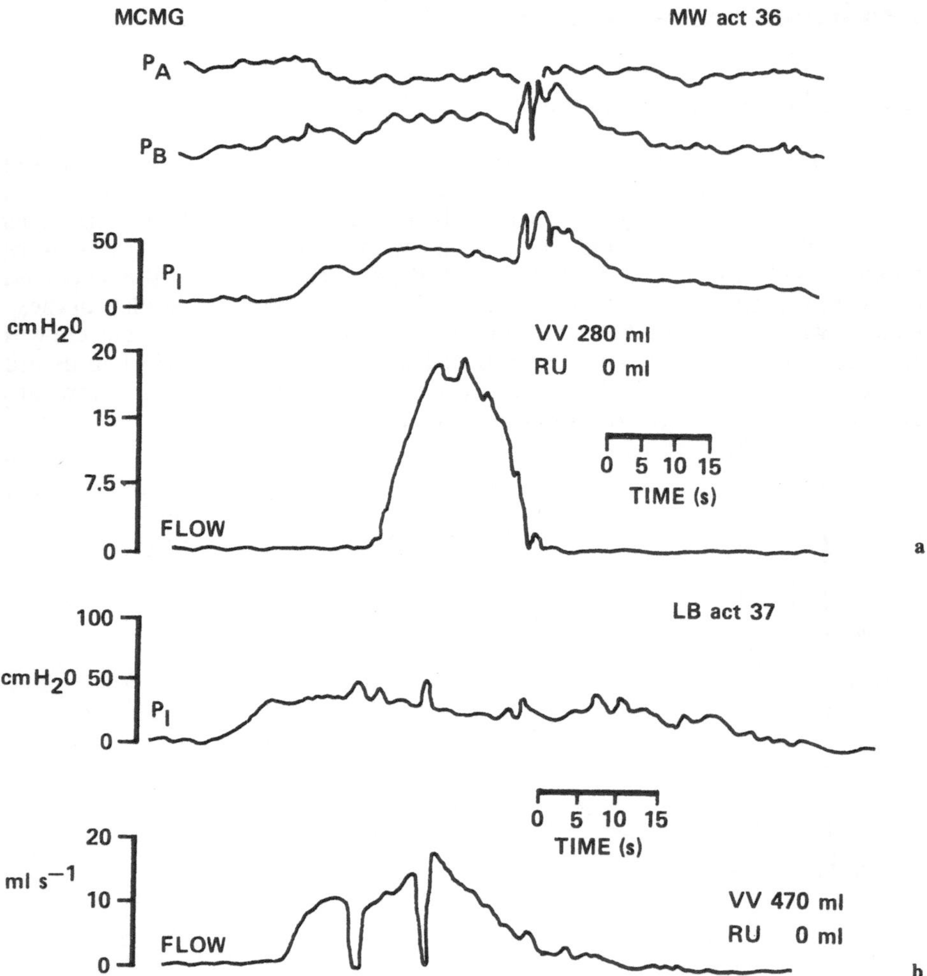

Fig. 17.3. Prostatodynia. Pressure–flow trace in patient of **a** 36 years, and **b** 37 years. Poor flow rate is *not* associated with raised detrusor pressure as would be expected if true obstruction were present. Note slight isometric 'twitches' in **b** as voiding is temporarily interrupted by pelvic floor contraction due to urethral pain (see detrusor–sphincter dysynergia p. 160). *PA*, abdominal pressure; *PB*, total bladder pressure; *PI*, subtracted detrusor pressure (Pdet).

Observations in Anxious Bladder Syndrome

The urodynamic pattern first reported in 1979 has since been encountered regularly in the urodynamic clinic. The initial free flow rate is abnormal, usually being both prolonged and intermittent in type (Fig. 17.4). The character of the urethral pressure probably reflects heightened pelvic floor muscle tone, and a mean maximum pressure of 117 cm H_2O (range 88–148) was recorded in patients studied by George and Slade (1979), all values but one being over 100 cm H_2O. In this series, despite a persistent desire to micturate during filling,

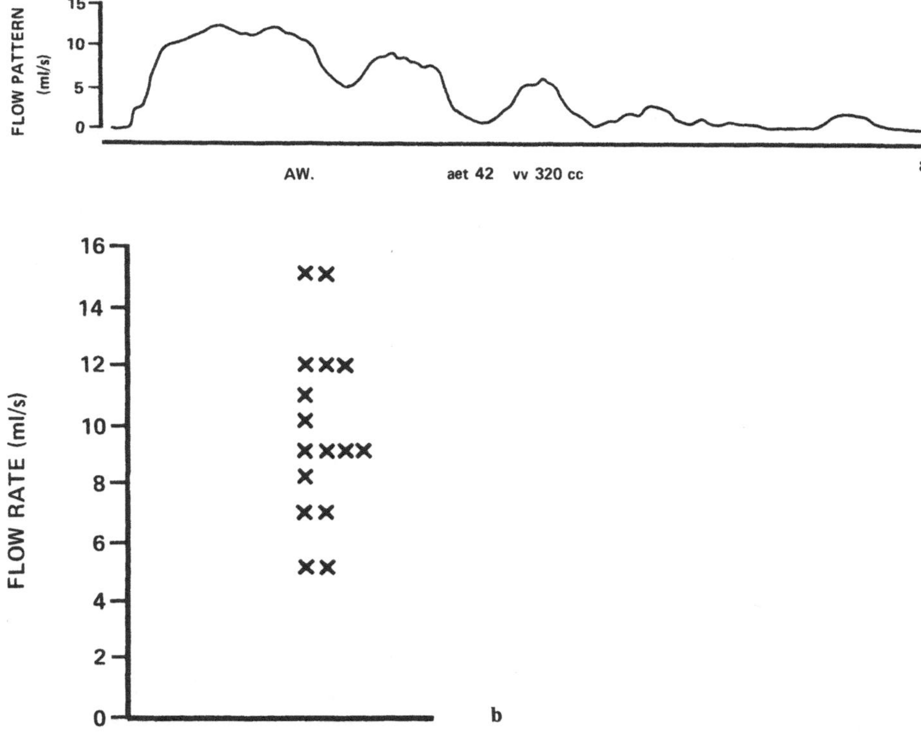

Fig. 17.4. **a** Typical flow pattern in anxious bladder syndrome. **b** Values of initial flow rate in 16 patients with anxious bladder syndrome (compare with Fig. 17.1c).

inflow cystometrograms remained stable and the mean capacity at the normal desire to void was 210 ml (Fig. 17.5). Micturition studies show the intermittent flow pattern to be the result of poorly maintained but synergic detrusor contraction waves (Fig. 17.6). Hesitancy of micturition, which is often severe in these cases, is due to a delay in the onset of detrusor contraction and to poor relaxation of periurethral muscle tone (Fig. 17.7).

Interpretation of Urodynamic Observations in Psychogenic Voiding Disorders

Urethral Closure Pressure

The urethral closure pressure in both prostatodynia and anxious bladder syndrome is undoubtedly well above the normal range when comparison is made with age matched controls (Abrams et al. 1983). This raised pressure may be due to increased tone of adrenergic smooth muscle, intrinsic urethral striated muscle (external urethral sphincter) or periurethral striated muscle (pelvic floor) or to a

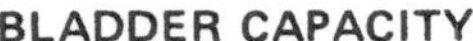

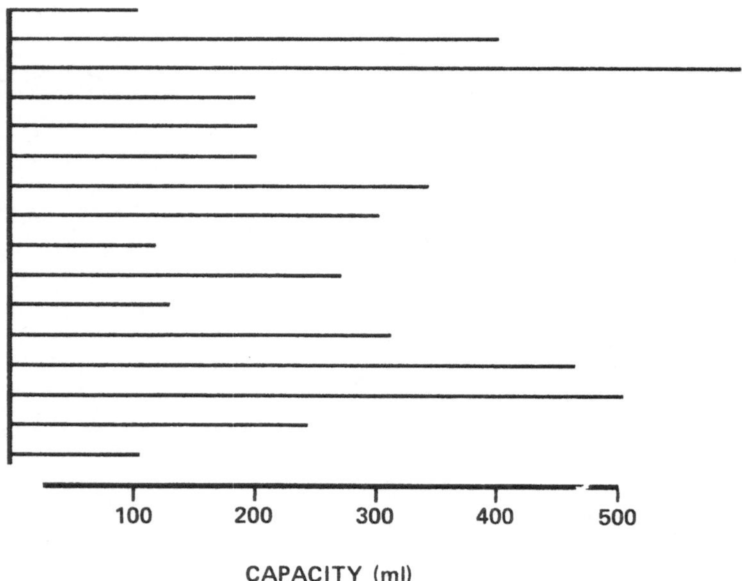

Fig. 17.5. Bladder capacity as determined by inflow cystometrogram in 16 patients with anxious bladder syndrome. Note that most patients request that filling be stopped prematurely as a result of excessive urethral sensation but some can be distracted and filled to a normal capacity.

combination of these components. The perineal pain experienced by patients with prostatodynia may be either the cause or the result of this increased muscle tone. However, some caution should be exercised before attributing the patient's discomfort to muscle spasm alone as similar values for maximum closure pressure are observed in patients with anxious bladder syndrome who complain more of frequency than local pain.

Inflow Cystometry

In patients with prostatodynia (Osborn et al. 1981) and anxious bladder syndrome (George and Slade 1979), inflow cystometry remains stable despite intense periurethral and lower abdominal discomfort. Bladder stability during the filling phase is typical of the sensory disorders and persists even when the bladder is over-filled ('superstable', p. 108). It would seem reasonable to propose that these patients possess a considerable capacity to inhibit detrusor contraction waves and this capability may prevent the onset of micturition (see below).

Voiding Cystometry

In patients with prostatodynia and anxious bladder the mean urine flow rates are low, and although many patients with prostatodynia do not complain of slow stream, values under 20 ml/s in this age group (mean age 42 years) should be regarded as abnormal (George 1985).

The cause of the low flow rate is attributable to a poor and often intermittent detrusor contraction which is particularly noted in patients with the anxious bladder syndrome (Fig. 17.6). Bladder outflow tract obstruction (high pressure/low flow) is not, therefore, present in these conditions and this observation explains the poor results obtained after transurethral surgery (Fig. 16.1, p. 141). Indeed it is often noted that the reflux of semen into the bladder, consequent upon this surgical procedure, frequently has adverse psychological effects on these introspective individuals. Andersen et al. (1980) in a study of younger men, some of whom presented with a low pressure/low flow urodynamic pattern, noted a satisfactory improvement after bladder neck incision. Mean post-operative flow rate, however, remained low (18.5 ml/s) in this series, a value considerably less than that expected for normal control men of a similar age and quite unlike the marked increase in flow rate which occurs following incision in patients in whom a true bladder neck obstruction is present (George 1985).

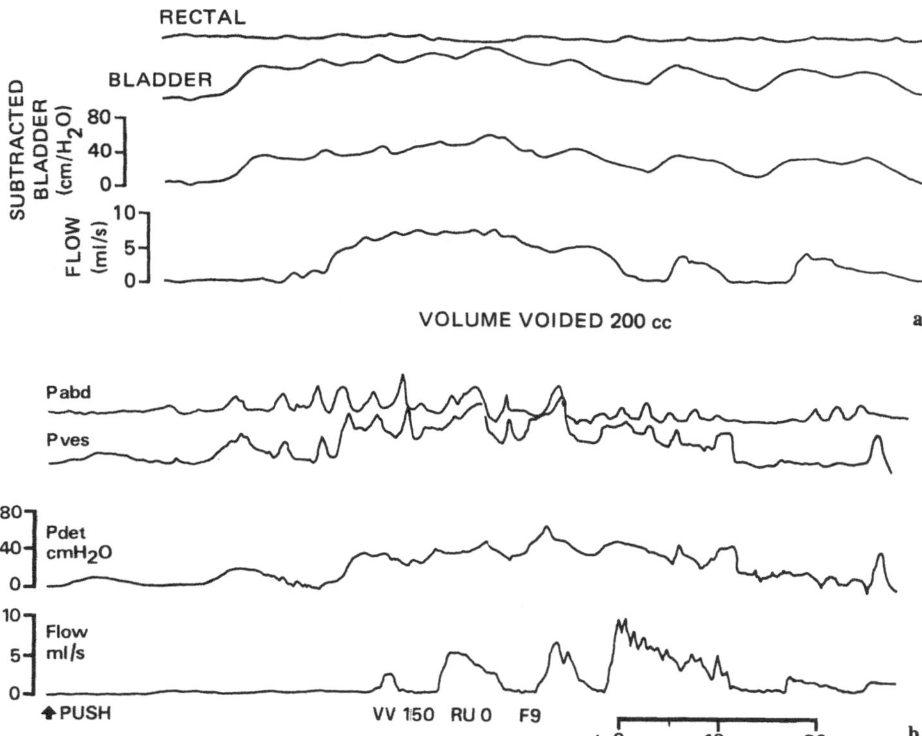

Fig. 17.6a,b. Micturition studies in anxious bladder syndrome. The poor and intermittent flow is seen to be due to a poorly maintained detrusor contraction. **a** patient aged 40; **b** patient aged 46. *Arrow*, patient commences attempt to void (instructed to assist flow by pushing). The pressure and flow relationship is synergic in both cases.

The aetiology of the voiding abnormality (Fig. 17.6) in anxious bladder patients remains unknown. One possible explanation is that over-inhibition of the micturition reflex might result from the anticipation of discomfort arising from a hypersensitive urethra during voiding. Dysuria is, however, relatively uncommon in these patients and it may be that the observed abnormalities are likely to be the result of neurological or psychological factors. Such conclusions are best deferred until specific histological and histochemical studies have positively excluded detrusor pathology.

The Underactive Detrusor and Chronic Retention

Paradoxically, despite the persistent urethral desire to void, patients with prostatodynia, anxious bladder and other sensory disorders demonstrate a remarkable facility for delaying micturition (O'Boyle and Parsons 1979). If asked to postpone micturition before urodynamic tests the patient may achieve bladder filling to normal or even supernormal capacity. Under these circumstances subsequent voiding may be prolonged and is often accompanied by the accumulation of residual urine (chronic retention) which, however, is usually passed at the next micturition (Fig. 17.7). This urodynamic behaviour is evident in the frequency/volume charts of these patients (see p. 144), which demonstrate an ability of the bladder to store adequate volumes of urine at certain times (e.g. at night or during periods of absorbing work).

The potentiality of the bladder to accumulate urine in association with inadequate detrusor contraction raises the possibility that such patients are at risk of developing chronic retention. It is generally assumed that painless retention usually results from longstanding infravesical obstruction causing detrusor muscle decompensation with subsequent overstretching of the bladder wall. However, cystometric studies on prostatic patients with high-pressure, low-flow obstructive voiding often demonstrate a low capacity, hypersensitive bladder (Abrams et al. 1979) and it is unusual to find large volumes of residual urine in such patients (George 1985). Webster et al. (1980) have suggested that,

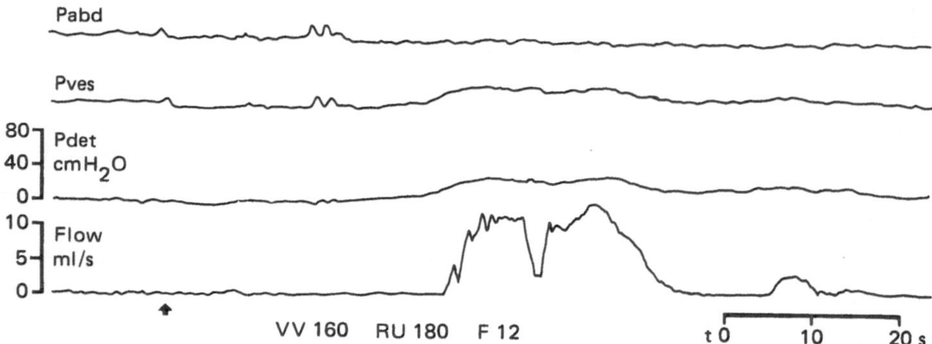

Fig. 17.7. Further example of severe hesitancy in patient with anxious bladder (30 s). On this occasion the patient was overfull and residual urine remained at the termination of micturition. (Dip in midflow curve largely due to flowmeter-induced artefact.) *Arrow*, start of attempt to void.

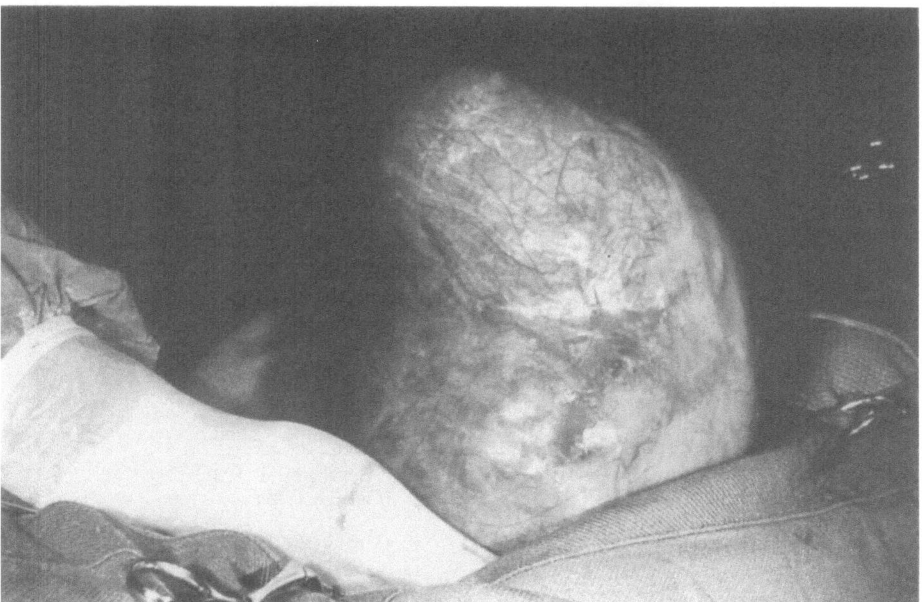

Fig. 17.8. Low pressure chronic retention. Large thin-walled bladder exposed prior to plication procedure. Urodynamics revealed underactive function with large volumes of residual urine. Some workers consider that this picture may be the end result of underactive detrusor states seen in younger men.

in contrast to the obstructive group, patients with weak or underactive detrusor contractions are more likely to develop painless retention which may eventually lead to the typical endstage thin walled 'atonic' bladder (Fig. 17.8; Webster et al. 1980). This hypothesis might have particular significance in those cases where an underactive bladder encounters additional resistance resulting, for example, from a prostatic adenoma which may commence to enlarge from middle age onwards (Franks 1954). However, although a tendency to gradual bladder enlargement may be detected over a period of years in younger patients with underactive detrusor muscles, the reduction of resistance resulting from outflow tract surgery which is commonly advised under these circumstances obscures the natural course of the dysfunctional process. It must also be acknowledged that such cases of chronic retention may be due to a neuropathy or myopathy which cannot presently be detected by routine clinical methods (Kirby et al. 1983).

Prostatodynia, Anxious Bladder and the Functional Disorders of Micturition

The spectrum of urological disorders which occurs in males under 45 years of age has been studied by Abrams et al. (1981). Some authorities have grouped the disorders together under the collective title of the 'functional' disorders of micturition (Siroky et al. 1981) (Table 17.1). On investigation most of these patients suffer from either detrusor instability or bladder under-activity, which in its most extreme form is described by Siroky as 'bladder areflexia with non-relaxing pelvic floor'.

Patients with poor detrusor contractions during micturition frequently have prostatitis-like symptoms and exhibit psychosocial and psychosomatic traits over extended periods of time (Siroky et al. 1981). The term 'bladder areflexia', introduced in an attempt to clarify the findings in these patients, is, however, questionable. This terminology should probably be reserved for those patients in whom a definite neurological lesion can be demonstrated. The inability to record a detrusor contraction during attempted micturition may occur as a result of either central or local inhibitory factors. In this context the presence of perineal electomyography needles and video cystometry cameras during urodynamic

Table 17.1. The 'functional' disorders of micturition in younger males without neurological abnormality[a]

Underactive detrusor states	(Abrams et al. 1981)
Low pressure/low flow dysfunction	(George 1985)
Bladder areflexia with non-relaxing pelvic floor	(Siroky et al. 1981)
Detrusor instability	
Bladder neck obstruction (high pressure/low flow voiding)	

[a] Three separate groups of patients may be included under this heading. Bladder neck obstruction (high pressure/low flow voiding) is a relatively uncommon condition. The majority of patients have symptoms due to either bladder instability or underactive detrusor (low pressure/low flow) dysfunction. Only the latter conditions are considered in this text which is concerned with the sensory disorders and these dysfunctions are given various titles by different groups of workers.

Table 17.2. Comparison of data from patients with prostatodynia (Osborn et al. 1981) and anxious bladder syndrome (George and Slade 1979). Normal data from author's series and Abrams et al. (1983)

	Normal	Prostatodynia[a]	Anxious bladder[a]
Number		22	16
Mean age (yr)		42	42
Mean maximal urethral closure pressure (cm H_2O)	80–90	121	117
Mean inflow cystometrogram (ml)	450–550	340	210
Mean subtracted detrusor voiding pressure, Pdet (cm H_2O)	60–70	34	42
Maximum flow rate (ml/s)	25–35	15	11

[a] The figures for maximum detrusor pressure and flow obscure the fact that the anxious bladder patients tend to have a more intermittent pattern of detrusor contraction than patients with prostatodynia (see illustrations above). The anxious group may merely represent an extreme variant within the spectrum of underactive detrusor function.

evaluation is unlikely to diminish the patient's general level of anxiety and contribute positively to the establishment of normal voiding dynamics.

It would seem reasonable in view of the urodynamic evidence presented in this chapter to propose that prostatodynia and the anxious bladder syndrome are closely related conditions in which the role of urethral hypersensitivity remains to be determined. Differences between the two may simply reflect the variable amount of psychological overlay that can be demonstrated in any group of patients. Symptomatically prostatodynia patients usually complain primarily of perineal discomfort and are less concerned with voiding disturbances. The anxious bladder patients, by contrast, exhibit urological symptoms mainly as an expression of their psychological difficulties. Urodynamic data are summarised in Table 17.2. There is no significant difference between the low pressure/low

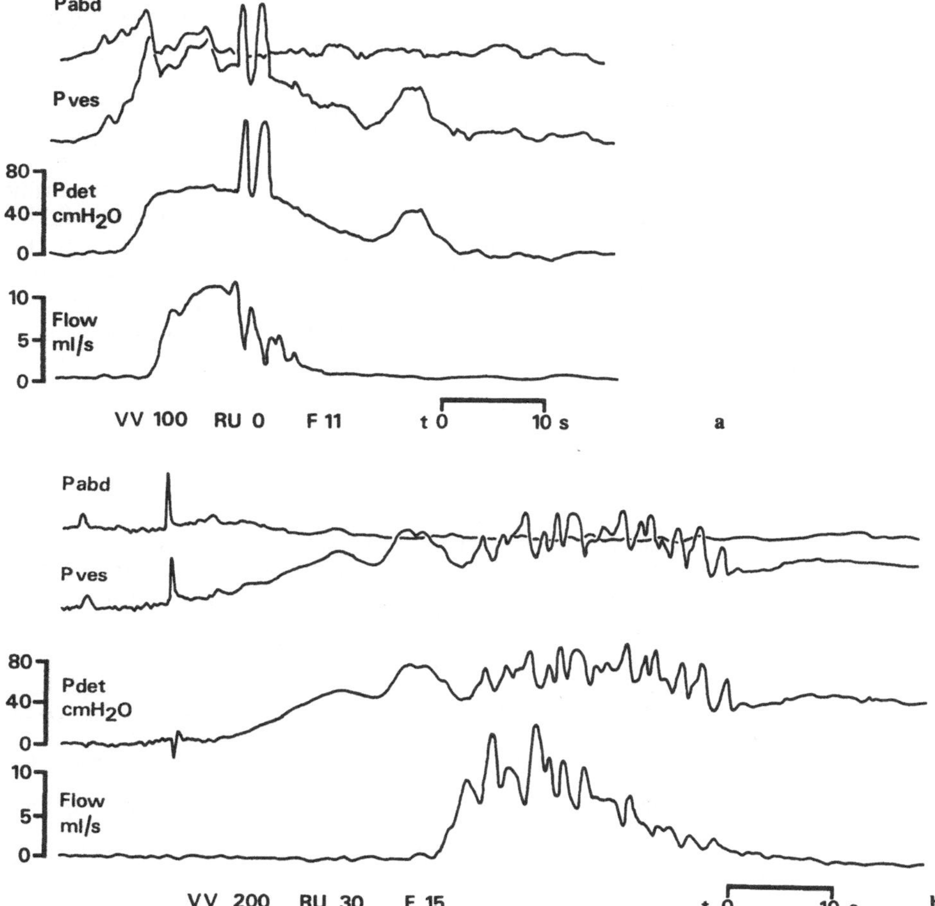

Fig. 17.9a, b. Two examples of micturating traces in prostatodynia where a voluntary interruption to the stream has occurred because of transient urethral pain. In both cases the dysynergic nature of the trace can be identified, the detrusor pressure rising as the flow rate falls (semi-isometric contraction). Compare these traces with the usual synergic form of voiding illustrated elsewhere in this chapter.

flow pattern observed in either disorder and in neither case is there any urodynamic evidence of outflow tract obstruction.

Low Pressure/Low Flow Micturition and Detrusor–Sphincter Dyssynergia

The poor and interrupted flow pattern present in many of the sensory disorders has led on occasion to the term detrusor–sphincter dyssynergia being applied to the form of micturition present in these patients. Careful inspection of the urodynamic traces, however, in both female (Fig. 13.3, p.109) and male (Figs. 17.3, 17.6) patients demonstrates that the diminution in flow generally occurs as a result of a fading detrusor contraction and this is an example of perfectly coordinated or synergic voiding.

Nevertheless, in some instances, detrusor and sphincter muscles may fail to work together, as when voluntary interruption is made to the stream by patients who fear or anticipate urethral pain (Fig. 17.9). It may therefore be physiologically correct to describe detrusor–sphincter dyssynergia as occurring under these circumstances although in the author's opinion this term should be reserved for those patients in whom a definite neurological lesion can be demonstrated. If the term is to be applied to sensory patients as described in this book it is important that an additional note should be made that the patients do not have neurological abnormalities that may be detected by clinical means.

References

Abrams PH, Farrar DJ, Turner-Warwick RT, Whiteside CG, Feneley RCL (1979) The results of prostatectomy; a symptomatic and urodynamic analysis of 152 patients. J Urol 121:640–642

Abrams PH, Shah PJR, Feneley RCL (1981) Voiding disorders in the young male adult. Urology 18:107–111

Abrams PH, Feneley R, Torrens M (1983) Urodynamics. Springer, Berlin Heidelberg New York, pp 48–61

Andersen JT, Nordling J, Meyhoff HH, Jacobsen O, Hald T (1980) Functional bladder neck obstruction—late results after endoscopic bladder neck incision. Scand J Urol Nephrol 14:17–22

Brown M, Wickham JEA (1969) The urethral pressure profile. Br J Urol 41:211–217

Drach GW, Binard W (1976) Disposable peak urinary flowmeter estimates lower urinary tract obstruction. J Urol 115:175–179

Franks LM (1954) Benign nodular hyperplasia of the prostate—a review. Ann R Coll Surg Engl 14:92–106

George NJR (1985) Lower urinary tract obstruction. In: Obstructive uropathy. O'Reilly PH (ed) Springer, Berlin Heidelberg New York

George NJR, Slade N (1979) Hesitancy and poor stream in neurologically normal younger men without outflow obstruction. Br J Urol 51:506–510

Kirby RS, Fowler C, Gilpin SA, Holly E, Kilroy EJG, Gosling JA, Bannister R, Turner-Warwick R (1983) Non obstructive detrusor failure. A urodynamic, electromyographic neurohistochemical and autonomic study. Br J Urol 55:652–659

O'Boyle PJ, Parsons KF (1979) Primary vesical sensory urgency; a clinical trial of bromocriptine. Br J Urol 51:200–203

Osborn DE, George NJR, Rao PN, Barnard RJ, Reading C, Marklow C, Blacklock NJ (1981) Prostatodynia—Physiological characteristics and rational management with muscle relaxants. Br J Urol 53:621–623

Siroky MB, Goldstein I, Krane RJ, (1981) Functional voiding disorders in men. J Urol 126:200–204

Stamey TA (1981) Prostatitis. J R Soc Med 74:22–40

Webster GD, Lockhart JL, Older RA (1980) The evaluation of bladder neck dysfunction. J Urol 123:196–198

Chapter 18

Application of Psychological and Psychophysiological Methods in Prostatodynia

C. Reading, P. King and H. Roberts

Introduction

The definition of a sensory disorder includes reference to 'perceived sensation' (p. 20) and supraspinal or psychological aspects of these conditions have been investigated by a number of workers, both in female patients with the urethral syndrome (Carson et al. 1980; Raz and Smith 1976), and in male patients with prostatodynia (Siroky et al. 1981). Personality traits characterised by excessive tension and neuroticism were considered by Segura et al. (1979) to be associated with an abnormal behaviour pattern in which habitual contraction of the pelvic floor muscles leads to persistence of the prostatodynia symptom complex. Anxiety, depression and hypochondria, reported on the basis of personality questionnaires, were the most common psychological abnormalities discovered in patients with chronic non-inflammatory prostatitis (Keltikangas-Järvinen et al. 1981). This form of analysis can be extended to include psychophysiological techniques which attempt to relate the subjective and behavioural aspects of affective and cognitive processes to quantifiable, objective measures obtained under controlled laboratory conditions. Similar techniques have been widely used in conditions such as depression, anxiety, schizophrenia, psychopathy and psychosomatic disorders (Venables and Christie 1975).

The most common psychophysiological test procedures are designed to assess the reactivity of the autonomic nervous system. Measures of palmar skin conductance and sweating have been shown to correlate strongly with skin-related sympathetic nervous activity (Wallin 1981). Additional information may be obtained from cardiovascular variables such as heart rate and finger pulse volume, recordings of respiratory excursion, and somatic measures such as the frontalis electromyogram. The response of these functions to an altered state of emotion or to changes in the level of arousal may be readily observed and recorded. 'Normal' and 'neurotic' groups are found to differ on various estimates of psychophysiological arousal, including basal activity, response amplitude, and the time taken for physiological recovery following an experimental stressor, which may be physical (e.g. the cold pressor test) or cognitive (e.g. mental arithmetic).

Procedure

Subjects

The study was carried out in two parts. In the first experiment a group of 20 subjects with prostatodynia (mean age 42 years) was compared with a small controlled group of 8 healthy subjects (mean age 29). In the second experiment a group of 24 subjects with prostatodynia (mean age 46) was compared with a controlled group of 16 subjects with bacterial prostatitis (mean age 39). The diagnosis of all patients referred for psychophysiological analysis was thoroughly verified by a previous passage through urological and urodynamic clinics.

Measures

The symptom distress check list (SCL–90) was used to assess neurotic symptomatology (Derogatis et al. 1973). This is a 90–item self-report questionnaire that assesses a broad range of symptoms commonly reported by psychiatric out-patients. The psychophysiological measures to be recorded were, in the first experiment, respiration rate, forehead EMG, heart rate and palmar skin conductance or sweating. In the second experiment, the measures were heart rate and forehead EMG. The laboratory assessment involved a 10-min adaption period after electrode attachment followed by a series of taxing procedures each of 2 min duration. These procedures were mental arithmetic, white noise of 90 dB intensity, two memory tests, a word recognition test and a reaction time test. Each test was preceded and followed by a 2 min base-line period.

The psychophysiological data were analysed as mean values for each of the 2 min duration session phases. Each function was measured to see if there was a significant overall difference between the groups and whether they reacted differently within the session. The statistical test was the analysis of variance with repeated measures. Each sub-scale of the SCL–90 was analysed separately using independent *t*-tests.

Results

In the comparison of patients with prostatodynia and normal control subjects there was a significantly higher mean heart rate for the prostatodynia group ($P=0.007$) and evidence of elevated frontalis muscle function, although this difference fell short of statistical significance because of a large within-group variability and the small number of subjects in the control group. Mean muscle tension levels within the patient group were similar to those obtained from patients with an anxiety state who had previously been assessed using the same procedure (Reading 1982). Respiration rate effects also differed between the two groups. The controls showed an overall decline in respiration rate at the end of the stressor session, which was not seen in the patients with prostatodynia, and this reduction in respiration rate is an example of the different recovery rates seen in 'normal' and 'neurotic' groups following exposure to stressors. Palmar skin conductance measures were similar for the two groups, possibly reflecting similar levels of alertness or arousal in response to the laboratory situation.

The prostatodynia group had a higher overall level of neurotic symptomatology on the SCL–90 with significantly higher (P=0.04) scores on the dimension of *somatic anxiety*, which contains 12 items relating to complaints of physical pain and discomfort. Scores on the dimensions of depression, general anxiety and hostility were elevated in the patient group but fell short of statistical significance. The remaining symptom dimensions did not differentiate between the groups. It should be noted that although the dimension of *somatic anxiety* is made up of questions regarding physical pain and discomfort it does not contain problems or symptoms specifically associated with prostatic or other urological disorders.

In the second experiment the symptom distress check list scores for the prostatodynia group were generally higher than those of the prostatitis group (Fig. 18.1). The highest mean score for the prostatodynia group was again on the somatic anxiety scale and there was a significant difference (P=0.05) from prostatitis patients, thus confirming the initial findings that patients with prostatodynia have generally higher levels of self-reported physical pain and discomfort, quite apart from any specific discomfort associated with the disorder itself.

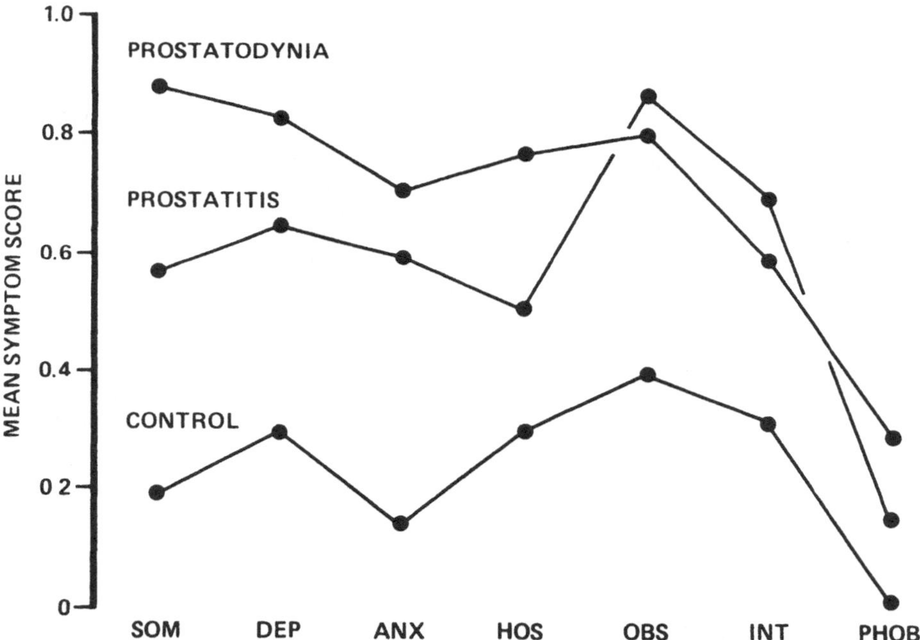

Fig. 18.1. Mean group scores on the symptom dimensions of somatic anxiety (*SOM*), depression (*DEP*), general anxiety (*ANX*), hostility (*HOS*), obsessive–compulsive traits (*OBS*), interpersonal sensitivity (*INT*) and phobic anxiety (*PHOB*).

Discussion

The two experiments suggest that patients with prostatodynia do have increased levels of self-reported, anxiety-related somatic discomfort and pain in comparison with those reported by healthy control subjects and patients with bacterial prostatitis. The symptom distress check list scores provide some support for the proposition that prostatodynia is associated with a general behaviour pattern of excessive tension while the physiological measures demonstrate that these patients are generally more aroused than those with prostatitis. The most marked differences between the groups were observed when measures of muscle tension and heart rate were made under challenging conditions such as mental arithmetic rather than during unstressed periods. It is therefore possible that, as suggested by Segura et al. (1979), the symptoms of prostatodynia are indeed related to pelvic floor spasm, which is secondary to a general overall activity of the skeletal musculature which occurs under stressful conditions. In particular, it is possible that an increased level of somatic preoccupation and anxiety, perhaps triggered during a period of discomfort of organic origin, may maintain a state of heightened tension following recovery from the initial complaint. Thus resolution of an organic prostatitis may be compromised by continuing muscle tension in the periprostatic region and pelvic floor of these patients.

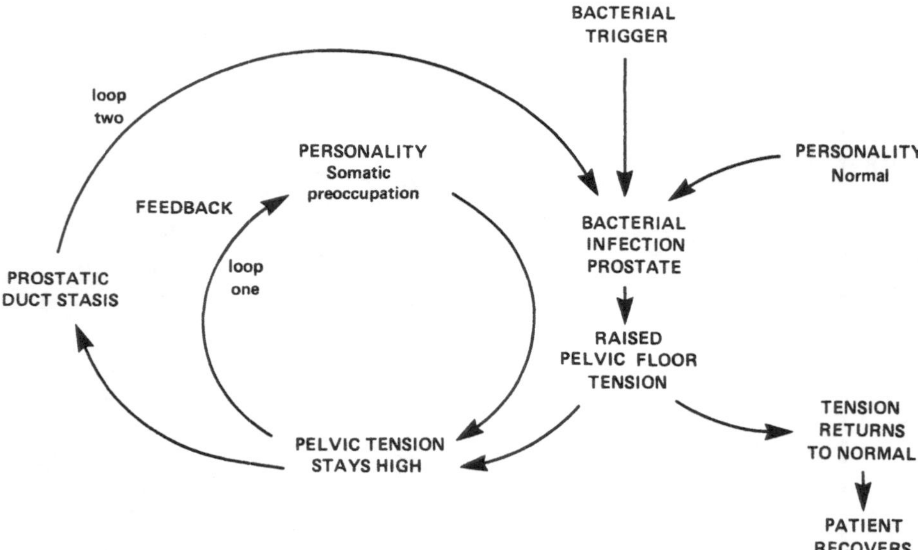

Fig. 18.2. Proposed course of events in psychosomatic voiding disorders. Following an infection of the prostate, local pelvic floor tension becomes raised due to local or reflex factors. Normal persons (*right*) recover and tension returns to pre-infection levels. Patients with excessive somatic preoccupation may be envisaged as entering a vicious circle of events. In *loop one* the patient becomes over-aware of the 'tension' in the pelvic floor and feedback leads to further preoccupation. In this situation no abnormality of expressed prostatic secretion might be expected. In *loop two* the excessive tension may predispose to duct stasis which could promote further inflammatory change within the prostate. Combinations of these two feedback loops might occur in many patients.

The patient may be seen as entering a vicious circle of events (Fig. 18.2). Firstly, the tendency to somatic preoccupation maintains a state of excessive muscle tension which of itself may be a cause of symptoms, and secondly the heightened tension with increased pressure in the prostatic urethra may predispose to further organic infection due to obstructive stasis and urinary reflux within the gland itself. Such a concept might explain the link between personality and disease and also illustrate why it is so difficult to obtain a cure in the prostatodynia patient.

It would be valuable to be able to predict those patients at risk of entering such a cycle of events. Almost half of the prostatodynia cases had abnormal levels of somatic preoccupation but this was also found in one in five of the prostatitis group. This finding in the prostatitis patients caused a reduction in the observed differentials between the two groups but raises the possibility that individuals with a combination of inflammatory disease and somatic preoccupation may be prone to a continuation of their symptomatology despite resolution of the initial inflammatory process. This interesting and important observation clearly requires further testing in a prospective clinical trial.

References

Carson CC, Segura JW, Osborne DM (1980) Evaluation and treatment of the female urethral syndrome. J Urol 124:609–610

Derogatis LR, Lipman RS, Covi L (1973) SCL–90: an outpatient psychiatric rating scale — preliminary report. Psychopharmacol Bull 9:13–27

Keltikangas-Järvinen L, Järvinen H, Lehtonen T (1981) Psychic disturbances in patients with chronic prostatitis. Ann Clin Res 13:45–49

Raz S, Smith RB (1976) External sphincter spasticity syndrome in female patients. J Urol 115:443–446

Reading C (1982) Experimental investigations of the psychophysiological basis of headache and its treatment using biofeedback. In: Main CJ (ed) Clinical psychology and medicine: a behavioral perspective. Plenum Press, New York

Segura JW, Opitz JL, Greene LF (1979) Prostatosis, prostatitis or pelvic floor tension myalgia? J Urol 122:168–169

Siroky MB, Goldstein I, Krane RJ (1981) Functional voiding disorders in men. J Urol 126:200–204

Venables PH, Christie J (eds) (1975) Research in psychophysiology. John Wiley, London

Wallin BG (1981) Sympathetic nerve activity underlying electrodermal and cardiovascular reactions in man. Psychophysiology 18:470–476

Chapter 19

Treatment of Prostatodynia and the Psychogenic Voiding Disorders

D.E. Osborn

Introduction

Numerous forms of therapy have been used in the past for patients with 'chronic prostatitis', many of whom would now be diagnosed as suffering from prostatodynia. Some of the treatment advocated appears bizarre in the light of today's knowledge, but still continues to be recommended by some clinicians. Thompson (1858) described the topical use of silver nitrate to produce blistering of the perineum as well as the application of leeches, both to perineal skin and to rectal mucosa overlying the prostate gland. Young et al. (1906) advocated urethral irrigation and prostatic massage, although the efficacy of either is indeterminate. Antibiotics have been frequently employed in prostatodynia with little or no response, which is not surprising in view of the complete absence of either infection or inflammatory change in the condition. As Stamey (1981) points out in his description of non-bacterial prostatitis, 'the use of those agents which are invariably ineffective simply adds credence to a non-existent infection which creates more anxiety for the patient, prolongs his misery and strengthens his concern that there must be an underlying mysterious infection which his physicians cannot cure'.

Although considerable advances have been made in recent years concerning the classification of inflammatory and non-inflammatory prostatic disease (Drach et al. 1978), similar progress has not, unfortunately, been made with treatment of the patient who is considered to be suffering from prostatodynia. However, the more objective studies described in previous chapters now afford an opportunity to define clearly the psychophysiological characteristics of the disorder and thereby to design a rational and progressive plan of therapy for this most troublesome condition (Fig. 19.1).

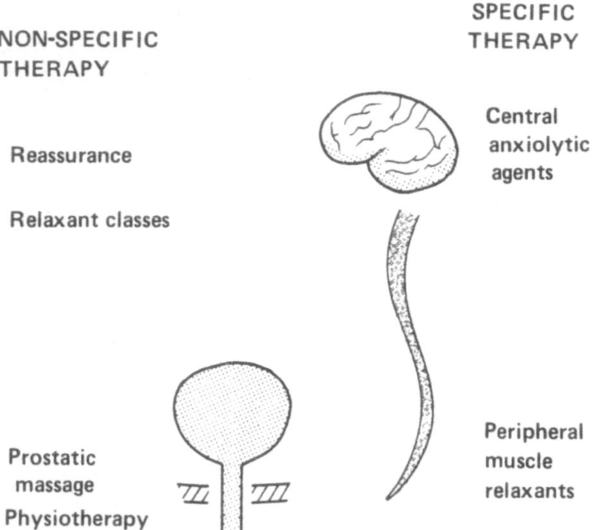

Fig. 19.1. Possible lines of therapy in the psychogenic voiding disorders.

Non-specific Methods of Treatment

Reassurance

The first duty of a physician treating a patient in whom the diagnosis of prostatodynia or anxious bladder has been made is to assure him that he does not have a serious disease. It is important that this reassurance carries conviction, especially as regards malignant disease, and it will always be troublesome convincing a patient that he does not have organic infection when he almost certainly will have previously received prolonged courses of antibiotics. For some patients simple treatments such as warm baths are effective and should not be overlooked; for those patients who complain of anal discomfort or bowel irregularity laxatives may be beneficial.

Prostatic Massage

This form of treatment has been used for years but has never been shown to have any positive therapeutic value. Such treatment, regularly performed on patients with a predisposition to somatic self-anxiety, might indeed do more harm than good. Massage is, of course, essential for the production of expressed prostatic secretion without which the diagnosis of prostatodynia cannot be made.

Physiotherapy

Local faradism or ultrasonic therapy to the perineum, though theoretically attractive, has not been found to be of value in patients with prostatodynia

(Osborn 1982, unpublished observations). Treatment with an ultrasound probe may invite similar criticism to that levelled at regular prostatic massage. Relaxation therapy used in combination with other non-specific treatment such as warm baths is advocated by Segura et al. (1979) as an effective method of reducing pelvic floor tension.

Antibiotics

Antibiotics can by definition have no therapeutic effect in view of the non-inflammatory, non-infectious nature of prostatodynia. If, however, there is any doubt about the exact diagnosis or the adequacy of previous antibiotic treatment, some authorities justify a final and full course of trimethoprim or erythromycin followed by a 3-month schedule with a urinary antiseptic (Blacklock 1982). This is to ensure as far as possible the eradication of any localised focus of infection within the gland.

Operative Treatment of Voiding Abnormalities

In the past, operative treatment in cases of prostatodynia has been performed with the intention of improving the urine flow rate (Fig. 16.1, p. 141). There can be little doubt, however, that transurethral surgery has been performed too often in these circumstances and the success rate for resections in all patients with 'chronic prostatitis' is only 30–50% (Stamey 1981). One reason for the failure of prostatic or bladder neck resection is that it is the peripheral moiety of the gland that is principally involved when infection is present. These parts of the prostate drain by ducts which empty below the level of veru montanum and this area is not usually resected during routine transurethral surgery. The principal reason, however, for the disappointing response to resection in true prostatodynia is that these patients do not have lower urinary tract obstruction, as is clearly described in Chap. 17. Resection is thus an illogical treatment (though difficult on occasion to resist) and patients rarely benefit from the procedure; indeed, anxiety may be made worse by subsequent disorders of ejaculation. The situation as regards transurethral resection of the prostate in patients with prostatodynia is not dissimilar to the position of gynaecological surgery in relation to pelvic pain. Twenty-five years ago Taylor (1957) remarked that 'premature resort to surgery is a characteristic error in the present day management of pelvic pain'.

Pharmacological Relaxation Therapy

Better understanding of the physiological and psychophysiological abnormalities in these patients has led to a search for effective relaxant therapy which might break the vicious circle of spasm and duct reflux referred to in Chap. 18. Hypothetically, it should be possible to obtain either central or peripheral relaxant effects by the use of the appropriate pharmacological agent.

Central Anxiolytic Agents

The best known agent of this type for the treatment of prostatodynia is diazepam (Valium, Roche), which also has some striated muscle relaxant properties. Unwanted drowsiness may well be a troublesome side effect of this drug, bearing in mind the mean age of the patients, but success at least in the short term has been reported by some authorities (Siroky et al. 1981).

Peripheral (Local) Muscle Relaxants

Much interest has centred on the use of pharmacological agents that specifically relax muscle thought to be important in the aetiology of the prostatodynia symptom complex. The bladder neck and pre-prostatic urethra of the male consists of a circular collar of smooth muscle which extends to surround the proximal urethra and is supplied by a rich plexus of sympathetic noradrenergic nerve terminals (Gosling et al. 1977). These fibres are intimately connected to muscle bundles which form the prostatic capsule and which are additionally found within the stroma surrounding prostatic acini (Fig. 19.2). Stimulation of sympathetic nerves during intercourse causes contraction of the smooth muscle bundles, leading to the ejaculation of prostatic fluid into and along the urethra, whilst retrograde transmission is prevented by simultaneous contraction of fibres in the pre-prostatic and bladder neck sphincter zones. Pharmacological blockade by appropriate agents might, therefore, be expected to reduce tension within prostatic ducts as well as lowering pressure at the level of the bladder neck. Unfortunately the scientific logic of such forms of treatment is offset to a certain extent by unwanted side-effects of the blocking agents, which in many instances restrict their clinical usefulness.

Relaxant Therapy for Post-micturition Dribble

Premature closure of the bladder neck following voiding with consequent 'trapping' of urine within the prostatic urethra is thought to be the main aetiological factor in this form of incontinence. Particularly satisfactory resolution of symptoms has been found in this group following treatment with phenoxybenzamine, which has been observed to relax the internal sphincter, thus permitting effective 'milk-back' following micturition (Osborn 1982, unpublished observations). The physician will be aware that the often fastidious nature of these patients leads to exaggeration of the degree of urine loss and routine advice concerning unhurried voiding will not be misplaced.

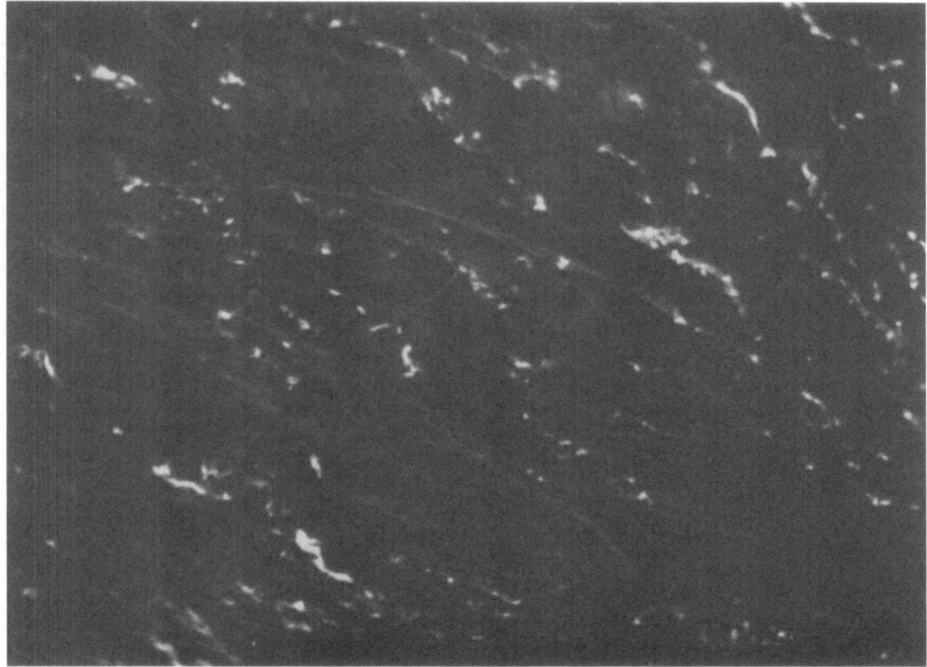

Fig. 19.2. Noradrenaline-containing nerve fibres (white beaded structures) ramify amongst the fibromuscular stroma of the male bladder neck. Note the faint autofluorescence of connective tissue elements. ×250

Relaxant Therapy for Prostatic Discomfort

Adrenergic Blocking Agents

The alpha adrenergic blocking agent phenoxybenzamine is known to reduce the amplitude of the urethra pressure profile by its action on the adrenergic musculature within the urethra (Donker et al. 1972) and has consequently been used to improve bladder emptying in patients with benign prostatic hypertrophy (Caine et al. 1981) and spinal cord injury (Sunder et al. 1978). In view of the urodynamic and neurohistological findings, phenoxybenzamine therapy should theoretically be of use in patients with prostatodynia. In a double-blind prospective trial, 13 of 27 patients reported a satisfactory symptomatic response after treatment with 10 mg nocte for 3 days and 10 mg twice daily for 1 month (P=0.027). Urodynamic evaluation, however, did not reveal any significant change although a non-specific increase in flow rate was noted in all arms of the trial (Osborn et al. 1981).

At longer term follow-up (median interval 10 months) 8 of 13 patients considered themselves completely cured and had ceased taking all medication. Two further patients were considerably improved but the persistence of minor symptoms necessitated continued follow-up (Osborn 1982, unpublished observations). This response rate, though by no means spectacular, represents a significant improvement over other therapeutic modalities tried to date in this most difficult group of patients.

Phenoxybenzamine is a potent adrenergic blocking agent and some side-effects of lethargy and dizziness are to be expected, particularly in older patients. For this reason the drug is recommended at a dose of 10 mg alternate nights for 1 week followed by 10 mg nightly for those occasional patients over 60 years old. This caution is necessary as the half-life of phenoxybenzamine is 24 hours. Younger patients, by contrast, tolerate a dose of 10 mg twice daily without difficulty, the main reported side-effect being a failure of ejaculation. Relief of pain, however, generally more than compensates for this loss which will be restored when therapy is discontinued. Naturally it is very important that the over-anxious patient receives a careful explanation of these reversible side-effects before therapy is commenced.

Striated Muscle Blocking Agents

Striated muscle relaxants such as baclofen (Lioresal) are generally prescribed for patients with spasm of skeletal muscle. This agent has been shown to facilitate voiding in spinal injury patients with detrusor–sphincter dyssynergia by means of a reduction in urethral pressure (Florante et al. 1980) and Osborn et al. (1981) showed baclofen to have a satisfactory clinical response in 10 of 27 (37%) patients with prostatodynia at a dose of 5 mg 3 times daily. At longer term follow-up, however, this initial response was not maintained, only three patients considering their clinical condition to be satisfactory.

The side-effects of baclofen in this double-blind trial were minimal and for this reason the drug was preferred by many older patients and hence remains a valuable therapeutic alternative to phenoxybenzamine in the patient who for any reason is unable to tolerate alpha adrenergic blocking agents.

Summary

The treatment of the patient with proven prostatodynia will involve the expenditure of considerable effort by the clinician, who must be aware of the complex psychological background to the cases and the inadvisability of resorting to illogical medical or surgical treatment regimes.

The rational approach outlined in this chapter enables the sympathetic physician to support and eventually discharge the majority of patients from his specialist care. However, it is unfortunately true that despite every effort a number of these patients will never consider themselves cured and will pursue an endless search for the medical opinion which can ease the burden of their discomfort.

References

Blacklock NJ (1982) Prostatitis: pathogenesis, clinical features and management. In: Recent advances in urology/andrology No. 3. Hendry WF (ed) Churchill Livingstone, Edinburgh, pp 185–197

Caine M, Perlberg S, Shapiro A (1981) Phenoxybenzamine for benign prostatic obstruction. Urology 17:542–546

Donker PJ, Ivanovic F, Noach EJ (1972) Analyses of the urethral pressure profile by means of electromyography and administration of drugs. Br J Urol 44:180–193

Drach GW, Fair WR, Meares EM, Stamey TA (1978) Classification of benign diseases associated with prostatic pain; prostatitis or prostatodynia? J Urol 120:266

Florante JL, Martin BF, Sporer A (1980) Baclofen in the treatment of detrusor-sphincter dyssynergia in spinal cord injury patients. J Urol 124:82–84

Gosling JA, Dixon JS, Lendon RG (1977) The autonomic innervation of the human male and female bladder neck and proximal urethra. J Urol 118:302–305

Osborn DE, George NJR, Rao PN, Barnard RJ, Reading C, Marklow C, Blacklock NJ (1981) Prostatodynia—physiological characteristics and rational management with muscle relaxants. Br J Urol 53:621–623

Segura JW, Opitz JL, Greene LF (1979) Prostatosis, prostatitis or pelvic floor tension myalgia? J Urol 122:168–169

Siroky MB, Goldstein I, Krane RJ (1981) Functional voiding disorders in men. J Urol 126:200–204

Stamey TA (1981) Prostatitis. J R Soc Med 74:22–40

Sunder GS, Parsons KF, Gibbon NOK (1978) Outflow obstruction in neuropathic bladder dysfunction: The neuropathic urethra. Br J Urol 50:190–199

Taylor HC (1957) The problem of pelvic pain. In: Progress in gynaecology, vol 3, Grune and Stratton, New York, p 91

Thompson H (1858) The enlarged prostate. Churchill, London

Young HH, Geraghty JT, Stevens AR (1906) Chronic prostatitis. Johns Hopkins Hospital Reports 13, pp 272–341

Subject Index